Clinicians' Guide to
Sleep Medicine

Clinicians' Guide to Sleep Medicine

Neil J. Douglas
Professor of Respiratory and Sleep Medicine,
University of Edinburgh,
Director of the Scottish National Sleep Laboratory,
Royal Infirmary,
Edinburgh, UK

A member of the Hodder Headline Group
LONDON • NEW YORK • NEW DELHI

First published in Great Britain in 2002 by
Arnold, a member of the Hodder Headline Group,
338 Euston Road, London NW1 3BH

http://www.hoddereducation.co.uk

Distributed in the United States of America by
Oxford University Press Inc.,
198 Madison Avenue, New York, NY10016
Oxford is a registered trademark of Oxford University Press

Whilst the advice and information in this book are believed to be true and accurate at the
date of going to press, neither the author nor the publisher can accept any legal
responsibility or liability for any errors or omissions that may be made. In particular (but
without limiting the generality of the preceding disclaimer) every effort has been made to
check drug dosages; however it is still possible that errors have been missed. Furthermore,
dosage schedules are constantly being revised and new side-effects recognized. For these
reasons the reader is strongly urged to consult the drug companies' printed instructions
before administering any of the drugs recommended in this book.

British Library Cataloguing in Publication Data
A catalogue record for this book is available from the British Library

Library of Congress Cataloging-in-Publication Data
A catalog record for this book is available from the Library of Congress

ISBN-10: 0 340 74205 4
ISBN-13: 978 0 340 74205 1

2 3 4 5 6 7 8 9 10

Commissioning Editor: Joanna Koster
Production Editor: Jasmine Brown
Production Controller: Bryan Eccleshall
Cover Designer: Terry Griffiths

Typeset in 11/13pt Adobe Garamond by Phoenix Photosetting, Chatham, Kent
Printed and bound in Malta by Gutenberg Press Ltd

What do you think about this book? Or any other Arnold title?
Please send your comments to www.hoddereducation.co.uk

Contents

Preface

The last 30 years have seen the medical aspects of sleep move from the realm of psychiatrists and psychologists into mainstream medicine. Sleep apnoea has been recognized as a common and treatable disorder affecting large numbers of people, the molecular mechanisms of narcolepsy are being unravelled and better treatments for insomnia developed.

In many countries training in sleep medicine remains relatively rudimentary and so reading simple up-to-date texts forms a critical part of training and of continuing medical education. This book aims to provide practising clinicians with a concise yet thorough understanding of sleep disorders. I hope that I have succeeded in conveying some of my enthusiasm for clinical sleep medicine, a field where doctors can genuinely transform their patients' quality of life by appropriate diagnosis and treatment.

The book is arranged by the common clinical presentations, sleepiness, difficulty sleeping, problems during sleep and then sleep in other illnesses. I have avoided following formal classifications of sleep disorders and side-stepped many standard but conservative approaches. I hope this has produced a book that is more readable and clinically useful.

I gratefully thank all my friends and colleagues who have both stimulated and helped me writing this book. These include Mike Fitzpatrick and Renata Riha for their comments. I particularly thank my family, Sue, Sandy and Kirsty for tolerating my long absences during the seemingly interminable gestation.

Introduction to sleep

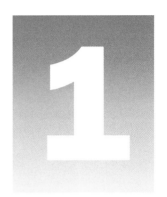

The importance of sleep

Sleep is vital to life; animals kept totally awake die in a few weeks.[1,2] Falling asleep at the wheel is the commonest cause of death on major highways[3] and sleep deprivation has been blamed for many major accidents at work including Chernobyl,[4] the *Exxon Valdiz* oil spill, the Three Mile Island nuclear plant and the Challenger Shuttle disaster.[5] Sleep problems are one of the most common reasons for consulting a doctor yet sleep histories are rarely taken[6] and sleep is barely taught in the undergraduate medical curriculum.[7] This book attempts to fill that gap by succinctly covering sleep medicine for the generalist while providing enough detail and references that the specialists may pursue their interests in depth.

Why we sleep

The function of sleep remains an enigma. Sleep occurs in all species and must have a vital role. Several theories have been proposed. One of the more likely is that it allows brain metabolic restoration. The rationale for this view includes the following.

- There are marked and reproducible EEG changes during sleep after sleep deprivation.[8,9]
- Sleep deprivation impairs cognition but has little effect on physical performance.[10,11]

This is compatible with the recent suggestion that sleep allows for remodelling of synaptic function.[12] This theory proposes that neural activity stimulates production of growth factors which may modify the pattern of synaptic stimulation within nearby groups of neurones. Sleep serves to decrease the activity in the previously active neurones and to permit this synaptic remodelling process to proceed efficiently. This theory also proposes that the locally produced factors resulting from synaptic activity may themselves promote sleep.[12]

Other theories have been suggested including that sleep:

- exists to conserve energy, but as energy consumption is only around 10 per cent lower during sleep this seems an unlikely explanation for such a ubiquitous process
- is a method of enforcing immobility to make animals less liable to attack by predators. This seems unlikely as species without known predators sleep, and predators are usually inactive when their prey is asleep.

How much sleep do we need?

Sleep requirements vary between individuals. Normal sleep durations in the UK are approximately 6.5–8.5 hours per week night, with slightly longer at weekends.[13,14] Some feel modern society sleeps too little[15] and there is no doubt that artificial light has made a vast difference to sleeping habits in recent centuries. If subjects are restricted to simulated natural winter lighting for a month, the average sleep duration rises from 7.2 to 8.2 hours a night.[16] However, there is no conclusive evidence that the usual 6.5–8.5 hours sleep is insufficient for most people.

Sleeping up to 10 hours a night did not significantly improve either subjective or objective sleepiness in 10 subjects but there was a minor improvement in vigilance.[17] On the other hand, 10-hour sleep opportunities improved sleepiness and performance in 12 subjects who usually slept for seven hours a night and fell asleep rapidly at baseline but had little if any effect on 12 subjects who usually slept for 7.6 hours a night.[18] Both these studies lacked control groups. However, the benefits of sleep extension for a sleepy subgroup were confirmed in a two-week study in comparison to subjects in a control group who continued their normal sleep regime.[19] Thus there are subjects for whom seven hours sleep per night is insufficient for optimal performance.

On the other hand, reducing sleep below the 6.5–8-hour range has definite effects. Thirty minutes less sleep per night may make one feel sleepy.[20] Reducing nocturnal sleep time to five hours a night results in subjective sleepiness and impaired mood after one night[21] and objective impairment of vigilance and performance after two nights.[21,22] Sleep reduction has greatest effects on cognition and speed of performance.[23,24] Subjects sleeping on average less than five hours a night function below the 95th percentile for performance of the non-sleep-deprived, according to a meta-analysis.[23] There are many anecdotes about individuals coping for long periods on four or five hours sleep per night – so-called core sleep[25] – and functioning satisfactorily. However, the evidence is that decision-making, vigilance and the ability to perform complex tasks will all be impaired at this level of sleep deprivation. Indeed, most of the subjects of these anecdotes have also been reported to fall asleep in boring meetings, indicating they were not after all superhuman.

What causes sleep?

The sleep–wake cycle is primarily driven by two processes. These are:

- A circadian component driven by the circadian clock in the suprachiasmatic nucleus (Chapter 7) which operates on a 24-hour cycle and causes maximal sleepiness in the afternoon and in the early hours of the morning. This has been called Process C – for circadian.
- A sleep drive which is dependent on the duration of previous wakefulness and the duration and quality of the last sleep.[26] This is sometimes referred to as Process S – the homeostatic drive for sleep.

The resultant balance between sleep and wakefulness involves several control mechanisms.

NEURAL MECHANISMS

Wakefulness is an active process maintained by activity of the ascending reticular activating system (RAS) originating in the pons and mid-brain.[27] The RAS may activated the cortex by two pathways; the ventral pathway projects to the hypothalamus, subthalamus and forebrain before diffusely radiating over the cortex, the dorsal pathway goes to the thalamus and then to the cortex (Figure 1.1).[28] The RAS controls the thalamic gate to incoming sensory information. During wakefulness, the reticular activating system depolarizes the thalamic reticular neurones permitting onward transmission of sensory information and thus desynchronized cortical activation.[29] Sleep is associated with inhibition of the reticular activating system allowing thalamic reticular repolarization, inhibition of onwards transmission of sensory information and thus uninterrupted synchronized cortical activity.[30]

The neurochemical systems promoting wakefulness via the ascending reticular system include:

- Noradrenergic neurones in the locus ceruleus in the pons which are continuously active during wakefulness but much less so during non-REM sleep.[31] Their efferents connect to thalamic relay neurones and to the cortex.

Figure 1.1
Schematic diagram of the asecending reticular activating system arising in the pons and mid-brain. The dorsal pathway projects to the thalamus and then diffusely to the cortex; the ventral to the hypothalamus, subthalamus and the forebrain then diffusely to the cortex. (Adapted from Bassetti and Aldrich,[28] with permission.)

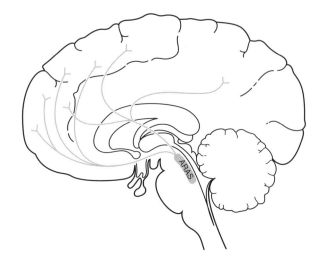

- Serotinergic neurones in the dorsal raphe nuclei which are most active during wakefulness and much less so during sleep.[32]
- Dopaminergic neurones in the ventral tegmentum of the mid-brain are involved in arousal and the maintenance of wakefulness.[33]

Sleep has conventionally been divided into rapid eye movement (REM) and non-rapid eye movement (non-REM) sleep since the observation by Aserinsky and Kleitman in 1953 that sleep was interspersed with regular periods of eye movement.[34]

Non-REM sleep onset is associated with altered activity in the ascending reticular activation system, the thalamus and basal forebrain. Stimulation of these areas induces sleep, whereas their ablation decreases sleep.[35] During light sleep, thalamic relay neurones show a combination of slow variations in membrane potential and superimposed 7–14 Hz bursts of spikes. These bursts cause excitatory post-synaptic potentials on cortical neurones resulting in the sleep spindles seen on the EEG. As non-REM sleep deepens the thalamic reticular neurones progressively hyperpolarize resulting in a reduction in sleep spindles and increased delta wave activity. Slow wave sleep is associated with increased GABAergic activity which both inhibits the reticular activating system and promotes the thalamocortical burst activity that causes slow waves.[36]

REM sleep is generated in the pons and cholinergic neurones in the anterodorsal tegmentum of the pons are critical to this process.[37] REM is associated with inhibition of the serotinergic neurones of the raphe nuclei, the noradrenergic nuclei of the locus ceruleus and of dopaminergic systems; this inhibition may facilitate cholinergic activity,[38,39] so REM sleep can be viewed as an interaction between cholinergic activation and monoaminergic inhibition.[40] The muscle atonia typical of REM sleep[41] is caused by activation of pontine cholinergic nuclei lying close to the locus ceruleus.[42] This results in post-synaptic inhibition of spinal alpha motor neurones.[43]

Pontine–geniculate–occipital (PGO) spikes accompany the eye movements and other phasic events of REM sleep. PGO spikes result from bursts of firing of cells in the peribrachial area of the pons adjacent to the superior cerebellar peduncle. PGO spikes are stimulated by acetylcholine[44] and inhibited by serotonin.[45] REM sleep deprivation results in a rebound increase in PGO spikes.

CHEMICAL FACTORS

Several naturally circulating chemicals can induce sleep:

- IL-1β and TNF-α, both of which promote non-REM sleep and inhibition of either cytokine inhibits non-REM sleep.[46]
- Prostaglandin E_2 may inhibit sleep.[47]
- Adenosine promotes slow wave sleep,[48,49] an effect inhibited by caffeine – an adenosine receptor blocker.[50] Adenosine seems to slowly build up in brain extracellular fluid during wakefulness and to decrease gradually during sleep, leading to speculation that it may induce sleep physiologically.[51]
- Serotonin may facilitate sleep onset and slow wave sleep while lesions of the raphe serotinergic nuclei produce total insomnia in cats.[52]

The production of some of these factors may resulting from synaptic activity in neuronal groups. Thus this neuronal activity may promote sleep independent of brainstem mechanisms.[12]

Sleep stages

REM sleep periods occur about every 90 minutes throughout sleep and REM sleep periods last around 20–30 minutes, tending to be longer later in the night. REM sleep is characterized not only by intermittent horizontal eye movements but also by loss of postural muscle tone[43] and by variability in autonomic functions; REM sleep is not a homogeneous state. The frequency of eye movements in REM sleep varies markedly as does the depth of breathing and heart rate. Periods of REM with frequent bursts of eye movements are associated with markedly shallow and variable breathing[53] and with surges in heart rate.[54]

Non-REM sleep occupies most of sleep in adults. During non-REM sleep ventilation,[55] heart rate,[56] cardiac output and arterial blood pressure[56] all fall compared to wakefulness. The vascular changes[54,56] seem to result largely from increases in parasympathetic tone accompanied by a lesser fall in sympathetic tone with reductions in circulating adrenaline and noradrenaline.

Non-REM sleep can be divided electrophysiologically into four stages with distinct EEG criteria[57] (Figure 1.2). This is an arbitrary splitting into stages of a process which is a continuum and it is likely that computerized analysis will make this staging redundant in the medium term. However, it is currently the standard technique.

Figure 1.2
Electro-oculogram (EOG), electro-encephalogram (EEG) and electro-myogram (EMG) traces in wakefulness showing alpha rhythm on EEG and high EMG tone.

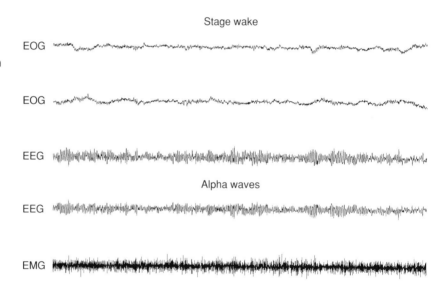

Those wishing to learn to score sleep expertly are referred elsewhere[57] but in broad terms these stages and wakefulness can be determined as follows.

Wake

The EEG is characterized by alpha rhythm with a frequency of 8–13 Hz (Figure 1.2) which is especially apparent over the occipital area. Alpha is present in approximately 90 per cent of normal subjects when resting with their eyes closed. Faster beta activity (14–25 Hz) is also often found, especially in frontal and parietal areas. As drowsiness starts, alpha slows and may vary in amplitude and may extend forward over the head, with beta activity becoming more prominent frontally. Slow rolling eye movements are a prominent feature of drowsiness.

Stage 1

The EEG changes from alpha to a low-voltage mixed-frequency pattern with the development of central theta activity (4–7 Hz) in association with slow eye movements on the EOG and gradual reduction of EMG tone.

Stage 2

Usually a few minutes after the onset of Stage 1 sleep, Stage 2 commences with the characteristic sleep spindles and K complexes. Sleep spindles are 0.5 to a few second runs of 12–14 Hz activity (Figure 1.3). Spindles are absent in Stage 1, most prominent in Stage 2 but may be seen in stages 3 and 4 sleep. K complexes are clear negative sharp waves which are immediately followed by a positive component, the whole complex lasting at least 0.5 seconds. The background EEG in Stage 2 is low-voltage mixed-frequency, but it is the occurrence of sleep spindles and K complexes which characterize the stage. The EMG shows tonic activity but at a lower level than in wakefulness. Slow eye movements may be evident early in the sleep period.

Stages 3 and 4

Stages 3 and 4 are often grouped together as either stage 3/4 or slow wave sleep (SWS) as both are characterized by the presence of high voltage slow

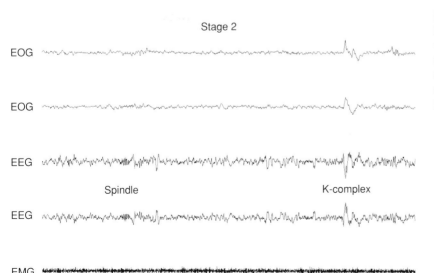

Figure 1.3

Neurophysiological signals (as in Figure 1.2) during Stage 2 sleep showing sleep spindle and K complex on the EEG and lowered EMG tone.

Figure 1.4
Neurophysiological signals
(as in Figure 1.2) during
Stage 4 sleep showing
delta waves on the EEG.

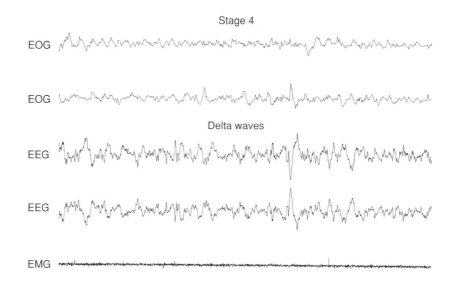

wave activity with frequency of 2 Hz or less. These delta waves occupy
(Figure 1.4) 20–50 per cent of the epoch in Stage 3 and over 50 per cent of
the epoch in Stage 4. In both stages slow eye movements are absent and the
EMG tone is reduced to a similar extent as in Stage 2.

REM sleep

The three characteristics of REM sleep are a desynchronized EEG, often
with sawtooth waves (Figure 1.5), marked reduction of EMG tone and
intermittent rapid eye movements on the EOG. The underlying EEG may
be similar to that in Stage 2 but the very low EMG tone and the presence of

Figure 1.5
Neurophysiological signals
(as in Figure 1.2) during
REM sleep showing
sawtooth waves on the EEG
and rapid eye movements
on the EOG.

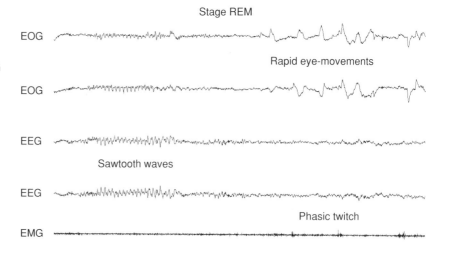

intermittent REMs usually allows easy differentiation. However, there may be several minutes of REM between eye movements and staging can sometimes be difficult, especially in real time.

The stages of sleep are summarized in Table 1.1.

Table 1.1
Stages of sleep

Sleep stage	EEG	EOG	EMG
Wakefulness	8–25 Hz	Variable	Normal
Stage 1	Low voltage	Rolling eye movements	Reduced
Stage 2	K complexes and sleep spindles	Absent	Reduced
Stage 3	25–50% high-voltage slow waves, –Hz	Absent	Reduced
Stage 4	More than 50% high-voltage slow waves, –Hz	Absent	Reduced
REM	Low-voltage fast-frequency sawtooth waves	Intermittent, jerky	Marked decrease
Movement	Unscorable due to increased EMG	Unscorable	Marked increase

AROUSALS FROM SLEEP

Brief awakenings from sleep, known as arousals, may be detected from the neurophysiological signals. Various different definitions have been used but the most common are:

- **American Sleep Disorders Association (ASDA) arousals** require a three-second or longer abrupt shift in EEG frequency to alpha or theta or >16 Hz, following at least 10 seconds of sleep, and if arising in REM there must be a rise in EMG tone.[58]
- **Rechtschaffen and Kales awakenings** require the dominant sleep stage of an epoch to be awake.[57] These wakenings are thus usually at least 15 seconds long.

Important simplifications about sleep stage distribution
In young adults:

- Sleep starts with non-REM.
- Non-REM and REM alternate approximately every 90 minutes.
- Slow wave sleep mainly occurs in the first third of the night.
- REM lasts longer in the last third of the night.
- Non-REM accounts for 75–80 per cent of the night.
- REM occupies the remaining 20–25 per cent.

FACTORS AFFECTING SLEEP PATTERN

Maturation

Sleep pattern changes with age (Figure 1.6).

Figure 1.6
Change in daily durations of total sleep and REM sleep with age.

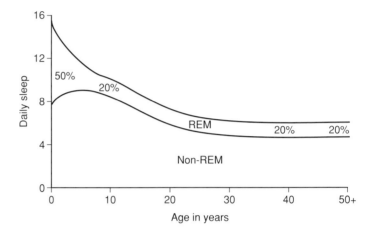

In infants

- Sleep often starts with REM sleep – called 'active sleep' in neonates.
- REM sleep may occupy 50 per cent of sleep.
- The REM/non-REM cycle has a shorter periodicity than in adults at 60 minutes.
- The EEG patterns of non-REM sleep are not fully developed until six months of age when slow wave sleep dominates.

In children:

- Slow wave sleep continues to dominate and is the main stage in the first third of the night. Awakening children from the first slow wave cycle may be almost impossible.
- The amount of slow wave sleep decreases progressively through the second decade to account for 15–20 per cent of sleep at the end of the teens.

In adults:

- Slow wave sleep progressively diminishes and is often absent in those over 60 years old.
- REM sleep is maintained into old age but declines in dementia.[59]
- Arousals from sleep increase markedly with age[60] (Figure 1.7).
- Sleep patterns vary markedly between elderly individuals.

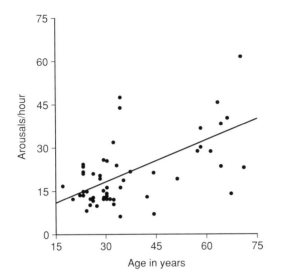

Figure 1.7
The frequency of ASDA arousals during polysomnography on normal subjects showing the increase in arousals with age. (Adapted from Mathur and Douglas,[60] with permission.)

Effect of sleep deprivation

Acute loss of sleep tends to result in:

- A rebound increase in slow wave sleep.
- A rebound increase in REM sleep occurs after slow wave catch-up has occurred.

Chronic loss of sleep tends to result in:

- Disturbance of the usual sleep stage pattern during catch-up. Thus, bizarre phenomena like early 'sleep onset'-REM (SOREM) sleep may occur.

Selective deprivation of either SWS or REM sleep results in a rebound increase in that sleep stage.

Exercise

Exercise results in marginally better sleep with small improvements in Stage 2 and slow wave sleep durations and an increase in total sleep time of around 10 minutes per night.[61,62]

Clinical features of sleep

Sleep onset is associated with hypnic jerks – brief and irregular limb twitches which are a normal phenomenon but occasionally cause concern to individuals or their bed-partner. During non-REM sleep there is regular breathing, slow rolling eye movements, decreased but still present muscle tone and preserved tendon reflexes. During REM sleep, breathing is irregular, jerky eye movements can often be seen through the eyelids and muscle tone is markedly reduced to the point of flaccidity. Particularly in neonates, myoclonic jerks involving the face and limbs may occur at irregular intervals during REM – these provided the label of active sleep instead of REM sleep in neonates.

Effects of sleep on human physiology

CENTRAL NERVOUS SYSTEM

Parasympathetic tone is increased in non-REM sleep, especially during slow wave sleep, whereas sympathetic tone tends to be decreased. In REM sleep there is marked variability of sympathetic activity.

CARDIOVASCULAR SYSTEM

These changes in autonomic tone in non-REM sleep result in a decrease in heart rate and cardiac output, with an associated 5–20 per cent fall in arterial blood pressure.[56,63] Sympathetic vasomotor nerve activity is increased and variable during REM sleep.[56] The swings in sympathetic tone result in marked variability of both heart rate and arterial pressure.[56] Sometimes bursts of eye movements may be preceded by a marked bradycardia.[64]

RESPIRATORY SYSTEM

Ventilation is decreased during non-REM sleep compared to wakefulness (Figure 1.8).[55] Breathing is very irregular in REM sleep where episodic severe hypoventilation occurs during periods with dense eye movements[53] (Figure 1.9). In periods of REM sleep associated with eye movements ventilation is around 84 per cent of that in wakefulness[55] but averaging the whole of REM sleep ventilation may be at around the same level as in non-REM sleep.[65] The hypoventilation is associated with a decrease in tidal volume with little change in respiratory rate.[55] This physiological hypoventilation during sleep is a major cause of the sleep related hypoxaemia found in patients with respiratory disease (chapters 9 and 11).

The upper airways narrow during sleep as the tone decreases in the muscles that dilate the pharynx[66] along with the sleep induced decrease in tone in other muscles. This results in increased resistance to airflow[67] during

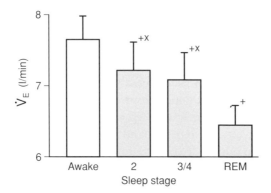

Figure 1.8
Ventilation in different stages of sleep. (Adapted from Douglas *et al.* (1982) Respiration during sleep in normal man. *Thorax*, 37, 840–4 with permission from the BMJ Publishing Group.)

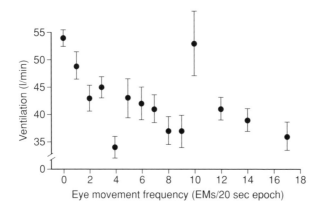

Figure 1.9
Relationship between ventilation and eye movement frequency in REM sleep in normal humans. (Adapted from Gould *et al.*,[53] with permission.)

sleep. In normal subjects the increase in upper airway resistance during sleep does not differ between the genders or with advancing age.[68] This increase in upper airway resistance during sleep contributes to snoring (Chapter 8) and obstructive sleep apnoea/hypopnoea (Chapter 2).

Hypoventilation during sleep is permitted by decreases in the ventilatory responses to both hypoxia and hypercapnia,[69,70] both of which are most marked in REM sleep. The ventilatory response to increased resistance is also blunted during non-REM sleep.[71]

GASTROINTESTINAL SYSTEM

The increase in parasympathetic tone results in decreased salivation and decreased gastric acid production during sleep. Both gastric emptying and intestinal transit are slowed by approximately 50 per cent.[72,73]

ENDOCRINE SYSTEM

Most hormones show cyclical variation in secretion. Some of these changes are under circadian control, for example cortisol, and are thus indirectly related to sleep, whereas others are directly under the control of the pattern of sleep, such as growth hormone and prolactin. Growth hormone production is closely linked to slow wave sleep and peaks during the first hour of sleep.[74] Prolactin levels start to rise around an hour after sleep onset and peak late in sleep.[75] Sleep inhibits TSH secretion.[76]

RENAL FUNCTION

During non-REM sleep there is decreased renal blood flow and glomerular filtration rate with increased water resorption and consequent decreased urine production. In REM sleep there is a further decrease in urine production.

Sleep and the clinician

Sleep problems are common. Approximately 10 per cent of adults report having significant problems with insomnia in the past year,[77–79] at least 20 per cent of bed partners are annoyed by snoring[80–83] and two per cent of adults have a medical cause for being pathologically sleepy.[82,84,85] Despite at least a third of the population being affected, most physicians do not routinely take sleep histories. Sleep histories were obtained in less than 20 per cent of patients attending outpatient clinics in one American study[86] and by no family practitioners in another.[6] Hospital doctors in the UK would almost certainly do worse than their American counterparts. Most medical schools teach little or no sleep medicine, with a median time of teaching on sleep in the British medical schools' clinical curriculum of two minutes for an activity which occupies around a third of human life.[7] Thus many doctors learn how to take a sleep history for themselves and often in a rather haphazard fashion.

As with any other area of history-taking, the questions asked will depend on previous responses but one North American way of remembering a reasonable list of topics is the mnemonic 'I Snored'. This stands for:

I   Insufficient sleep and insomnia

S   Snoring and shift work

N   Narcolepsy/cataplexy

O   Obstructive apnoea

R   Refreshing sleep
E   Excessive daytime sleepiness
D   Drugs – sedative and stimulant

Another mnemonic which may help with targeted physical examination in patients with possible sleep apnoea/hypopnoea syndrome is 'A snort', standing for:

A   Acromegaly/hypothyroid?

S   Systolic BP
N   Nose
O   Obesity
R   Retrognathia
T   Throat narrowed?

It is unimportant whether these mnemonics are followed provided these key areas are covered and built on as needed. Subsequent chapters will describe how to build on them to reach a diagnosis and plan management.

Useful reviews

- National Commission on Sleep Disorders Research. (1993) *Wake up America: A national sleep alert.* Washington: US Government Printing Office.
- Benington, J.H. (2000) Sleep homeostasis and the function of sleep. *Sleep*, **23**, 959–66.

References

1 Everson, C.A., Bergmann, B.M., Rechtschaffen, A. (1989) Sleep deprivation in the rat: III. Total sleep deprivation. *Sleep*, **12**, 13–21.
2 Rechtschaffen, A., Bergmann, B.M., Everson, C.A., Kushida, C.A., Gilliland, M.A. (1989) Sleep deprivation in the rat: X. Integration and discussion of the findings. *Sleep*, **12**, 68–87.
3 Horne, J.A., Reyner, L.A. (1995) Sleep related vehicle accidents. *BMJ*, **310**, 565–7.

4 Mitler, M.M., Carskadon, M.A., Czeisler, C.A., Dement, W.C., Dinges, D.F., Graeber, R.C. (1988) Catastrophes, sleep, and public policy: consensus report. *Sleep*, **11**, 100–9.

5 National Commission on Sleep Disorders Research. (1993) *Wake up America: A national sleep alert*. Washington: US Government Printing Office.

6 Haponik, E.F., Frye, A.W., Richards, B., Wymer, A., Hinds, A., Pearce, K. *et al.* (1996) Sleep history is neglected diagnostic information. Challenges for primary care physicians. *J. Gen. Intern. Med.*, **11**, 759–61.

7 Stores, G., Crawford, C. (1998) Medical student education in sleep and its disorders. *J. R. Coll. Physicians Lond.*, **32**, 149–53.

8 Webb, W.B., Agnew, H.W. (1975) The effects on subsequent sleep of an acute restriction of sleep length. *Psychophysiology*, **12**, 367–70.

9 Webb, W.B., Agnew, H.W. (1971) Stage 4 sleep: influence of time course variables. *Science*, **174**, 1354–6.

10 Horne, J.A. (1983) Human sleep and tissue restitution: some qualifications and doubts. *Clin. Sci. (Colch)*, **65**, 569–77.

11 VanHelder, T., Radomski, M.W. (1989) Sleep deprivation and the effect on exercise performance. *Sports Med.*, 7, 235–47.

12 Krueger, J.M., Obal, F., Fang, J. (2001) Why we sleep: a theoretical view of sleep function. *Sleep Medicine Reviews*, **3**, 119–29.

13 Tune, G.S. (1968) Sleep and wakefulness in normal human adults. *BMJ*, **2**, 269–71.

14 Tune, G.S. (1969) Sleep and wakefulness in 509 normal human adults. *Br. J. Med. Psychol.*, **42**, 75–80.

15 Bonnet, M.H., Arand, D.L. (1995) We are chronically sleep deprived. *Sleep*, **18**, 908–11.

16 Wehr, T.A., Moul, D.E., Barbato, G., Giesen, H.A., Seidel, J.A., Barker, C. *et al.* (1993) Conservation of photoperiod-responsive mechanisms in humans. *Am. J. Physiol.*, **265**, R846–R857.

17 Harrison, Y., Horne, J.A. (1996) Long-term extension to sleep – are we really chronically sleep deprived? *Psychophysiology*, **33**, 22–30.

18 Roehrs, T., Timms, V., Zwyghuizen-Doorenbos, A., Roth, T. (1989) Sleep extension in sleepy and alert normals. *Sleep*, **12**, 449–57.

19 Roehrs, T., Shore, E., Papineau, K., Rosenthal, L., Roth, T. (1996) A two-week sleep extension in sleepy normals. *Sleep*, **19**, 576–82.

20 Carskadon, M.A., Dement, W.C. (1981) Cumulative effects of sleep restriction on daytime sleepiness. *Psychophysiology*, **18**, 107–13.

21 Dinges, D.F., Pack, F., Williams, K., Gillen, K.A., Powell, J.W., Ott, G.E. *et al.* (1997) Cumulative sleepiness, mood disturbance, and psychomotor vigilance performance decrements during a week of sleep restricted to 4–5 hours per night. *Sleep*, **20**, 267–77.

22 Wilkinson, R.T., Edwards, R.S., Haines, E. (1966) Performance following a night of reduced sleep. *Psychonomic Sci.*, **5**, 472.

23 Pilcher, J.J., Huffcutt, A.I. (1996) Effects of sleep deprivation on performance: a meta-analysis. *Sleep*, **19**, 318–26.

24 Koslowsky, M., Babkoff, H. (1992) Meta-analysis of the relationship between total sleep deprivation and performance. *Chronobiol. Int.*, **9**, 132–6.

25 Horne, J. (1988) *Why we sleep.* Oxford: Oxford University Press.

26 Borbely, A.A., Achermann, P. (1999) Sleep homeostasis and models of sleep regulation. *J. Biol. Rhythms,* **14**, 557–68.

27 Moruzzi, G., Magoun, H.W. (1949) Brainstem reticular formation and activation of the EEG. Electroencephalogr. *Clin. Neurophysiol.*, **1**, 455–73.

28 Bassetti, C., Aldrich, M.S. (1996) Consciousness, delirium and coma, in M.S. Albin, (ed). *Textbook of Neuroanesthesia with Neurosurgical and Neuroscience Perspectives*, pp. 369–408. New York: McGraw-Hill.

29 Steriade, M., Gloor, P., Llinas, R.R., Lopes de Silva, F.H., Mesulam, M.M. (1990) Report of IFCN Committee on Basic Mechanisms. Basic mechanisms of cerebral rhythmic activities. *Electroencephalogr. Clin. Neurophysiol.*, **76**, 481–508.

30 Steriade, M. (2000) Corticothalamic resonance, states of vigilance and mentation. *Neuroscience*, 101, 243–76.

31 Jones, B.E. (1991) The role of noradrenergic locus coeruleus neurons and neighboring cholinergic neurons of the pontomesencephalic tegmentum in sleep–wake states. *Prog. Brain Res.*, **88**, 533–43.

32 Lydic, R. (1988) Central regulation of sleep and autonomic physiology, in R. Lydic and J.F. Biebuyck (eds). *Clinical Physiology of Sleep*, pp. 1–19. Bethesda, MD: American Physiological Society.

33 Bagetta, G., De Sarro, G., Priolo, E., Nistico, G. (1988) Ventral tegmental area: site through which dopamine D2-receptor agonists evoke behavioural and electrocortical sleep in rats. *Br. J. Pharmacol.*, **95**, 860–6.

34 Aserinsky, E., Kleitman, N. (1953) Regularly occurring periods of eye motility and concomittant phenomena during sleep. *Science*, **118**, 273–4.

35 Sallanon, M., Denoyer, M., Kitahama, K., Aubert, C., Gay, N., Jouvet, M. (1989) Long-lasting insomnia induced by preoptic neuron lesions and its transient reversal by muscimol injection into the posterior hypothalamus in the cat. *Neuroscience*, **32**, 669–83.

36 von Krosigk, M., Bal, T., McCormick, D.A. (1993) Cellular mechanisms of a synchronized oscillation in the thalamus. *Science*, **261**, 361–4.

37 Yamamoto, K., Mamelak, A.N., Quattrochi, J.J., Hobson, J.A. (1990) A cholinoceptive desynchronized sleep induction zone in the anterodorsal pontine tegmentum: spontaneous and drug-induced neuronal activity. *Neuroscience*, **39**, 295–304.

38 Hobson, J.A., McCarley, R.W., Pivik, R.T., Freedman, R. (1974) Selective firing by cat pontine brain stem neurons in desynchronized sleep. *J. Neurophysiol.*, **37**, 497–511.

39 Jones, B.E. (1991) Paradoxical sleep and its chemical/structural substrates in the brain. *Neuroscience*, **40**, 637–56.

40 McCarley, R.W., Hobson, J.A. (1975) Neuronal excitability modulation over the sleep cycle: a structural and mathematical model. *Science*, **189**, 58–60.

41 Jouvet, M., Michel, F. (1959) Correlations electromyographiques du sommeil chez le chat decortique et mesencephalique chronique. *C. R. Soc. Biol.*, **153**, 422.

42 Sakai, K. (1986) Central mechanisms of paradoxical sleep. *Brain Dev.*, **8**, 402–7.

43 Morales, F.R., Chase, M.H. (1978) Intracellular recording of lumbar motoneuron membrane potential during sleep and wakefulness. *Exp. Neurol.*, **62**, 821–7.

44 Baghdoyan, H.A., Rodrigo-Angulo, M.L., McCarley, R.W., Hobson, J.A. (1987) A neuroanatomical gradient in the pontine tegmentum for the cholinoceptive induction of desynchronized sleep signs. *Brain Res.*, **414**, 245–61.

45 Luebke, J.I., Greene, R.W., Semba, K., Kamondi, A., McCarley, R.W., Reiner, P.B. (1992) Serotonin hyperpolarizes cholinergic low-threshold burst neurons in the rat laterodorsal tegmental nucleus *in vitro*. *Proc. Natl. Acad. Sci. USA*, **89**, 743–7.

46 Krueger, J.M., Obal, F., Fang, J. (1999) Humoral regulation of physiological sleep: cytokines and GHRH. *J. Sleep Res.*, **8** (Suppl. 1), 53–9.

47 Krueger, J.M., Kapas, L., Opp, M.R., Obal, F. (1992) Prostaglandins E2 and D2 have little effect on rabbit sleep. *Physiol. Behav.*, **51**, 481–5.

48 Satoh, S., Matsumura, H., Hayaishi, O. (1998) Involvement of adenosine A2A receptor in sleep promotion. *Eur. J. Pharmacol.*, **351**, 155–62.

49 Satoh, S., Matsumura, H., Suzuki, F., Hayaishi, O. (1996) Promotion of sleep mediated by the A2a-adenosine receptor and possible involvement of this receptor in the sleep induced by prostaglandin D2 in rats. *Proc. Natl. Acad. Sci. USA*, **93**, 5980–4.

50 Benington, J.H., Kodali, S.K., Heller, H.C. (1995) Stimulation of A1 adenosine receptors mimics the electroencephalographic effects of sleep deprivation. *Brain Res.*, **692**, 79–85.

51 Porkka-Heiskanen, T., Strecker, R.E., McCarley, R.W. (2000) Brain site-specificity of extracellular adenosine concentration changes during sleep deprivation and spontaneous sleep: an *in vivo* microdialysis study. *Neuroscience*, **99**, 507–17.

52 Jouvet, M. (1972) The role of monoamines and acetylcholine-containing neurons in the regulation of the sleep-waking cycle. *Ergeb. Physiol.*, **64**, 166–307.

53 Gould, G.A., Gugger, M., Molloy, J., Tsara, V., Shapiro, C.M., Douglas, N.J. (1988) Breathing pattern and eye movement density during REM sleep in humans. *Am. Rev. Respir. Dis.*, **138**, 874–7.

54 Baust, W., Bohnert, B. (1969) The regulation of heart rate during sleep. *Exp. Brain Res.*, 7, 169–80.

55 Douglas, N.J., White, D.P., Pickett, C.K., Weil, J.V., Zwillich, C.W. (1982) Respiration during sleep in normal man. *Thorax*, **37**, 840–4.

56 Somers, V.K., Dyken, M.E., Mark, A.L., Abboud, F.M. (1993) Sympathetic-nerve activity during sleep in normal subjects. *N. Engl. J. Med.*, **328**, 303–7.

57 Rechtschaffen, A., Kales, A. (1968) *A Manual of Standardized Terminology, Techniques and Scoring System for Sleep Stages of Human Subjects.* Los Angeles, CA: UCLA Brain Information Service.

58 American Sleep Disorders Association (ASDA). (1992) EEG arousals: scoring rules and examples: a preliminary report from the Sleep Disorders Atlas Task Force of the American Sleep Disorders Association. *Sleep*, 15, 173–84.

59 Prinz, P.N., Peskind, E.R., Vitaliano, P.P., Raskind, M.A., Eisdorfer, C., Zemcuznikov, N. *et al.* (1982) Changes in the sleep and waking EEGs of nondemented and demented elderly subjects. *J. Am. Geriatr. Soc.*, **30**, 86–93.

60 Mathur, R., Douglas, N.J. (1995) Frequency of EEG arousals from nocturnal sleep in normal subjects. *Sleep*, 18, 330–3.

61 Youngstedt, S.D., O'Connor, P.J., Dishman, R.K. (1997) The effects of acute exercise on sleep: a quantitative synthesis. *Sleep*, **20**, 203–14.

62 Driver, H.S., Taylor, S.R. (2000) Exercise and sleep. *Sleep Medicine Reviews*, **4**, 387–402.

63 Bristow, J.D., Honour, A.J., Pickering, T.G., Sleight, P. (1969) Cardiovascular and respiratory changes during sleep in normal and hypertensive subjects. *Cardiovasc. Res.*, **3**, 476–85.

64 Taylor, W.B., Moldofsky, H., Furedy, J.J. (1985) Heart rate deceleration in REM sleep: an orienting reaction interpretation. *Psychophysiology*, **22**, 110–15.

65 White, D.P., Weil, J.V., Zwillich, C.W. (1985) Metabolic rate and breathing during sleep. *J. Appl. Physiol.*, **59**, 384–91.

66 Tangel, D.J., Mezzanotte, W.S., White, D.P. (1995) Influences of NREM sleep on activity of palatoglossus and levator palatini muscles in normal men. *J. Appl. Physiol.*, **78**, 689–95.

67 Hudgel, D.W., Martin, R.J., Johnson, B., Hill, P. (1984) Mechanics of the respiratory system and breathing pattern during sleep in normal humans. *J. Appl. Physiol.*, 56, 133–7.

68 Thurnheer, R., Wraith, P.K., Douglas, N.J. (2001) Influence of age and gender on upper airway resistance in NREM and REM sleep. *J. Appl. Physiol.*, **90**, 981–8.

69 Douglas, N.J., White, D.P., Weil, J.V., Pickett, C.K., Zwillich, C.W. (1982) Hypercapnic ventilatory response in sleeping adults. *Am. Rev. Respir. Dis.*, **126**, 758–62.

70 Douglas, N.J., White, D.P., Weil, J.V., Pickett, C.K., Martin, R.J., Hudgel, D.W. *et al.* (1982) Hypoxic ventilatory response decreases during sleep in normal men. *Am. Rev. Respir. Dis.*, **125**, 286–9.

71 Wiegand, L., Zwillich, C.W., White, D.P. (1988) Sleep and the ventilatory response to resistive loading in normal men. *J. Appl. Physiol.*, **64**, 1186–95.

72 Goo, R.H., Moore, J.G., Greenberg, E., Alazraki, N.P. (1987) Circadian variation in gastric emptying of meals in humans. *Gastroenterology*, **93**, 515–18.

73 Kumar, D. (1994) Sleep as a modulator of human gastrointestinal motility. *Gastroenterology*, **107**, 1548–50.

74 Sassin, J.F., Parker, D.C., Mace, J.W., Gotlin, R.W., Johnson, L.C., Rossman, L.G. (1969) Human growth hormone release: relation to slow-wave sleep and sleep-walking cycles. *Science*, *165*, 513–15.

75 Sassin, J.F., Frantz, A.G., Kapen, S., Weitzman, E.D. (1973) The nocturnal rise of human prolactin is dependent on sleep. *J. Clin. Endocrinol. Metab.*, **37**, 436–40.

76 Brabant, G., Prank, K., Ranft, U., Schuermeyer, T., Wagner, T.O., Hauser, H. *et al.* (1990) Physiological regulation of circadian and pulsatile thyrotropin secretion in normal man and woman. *J. Clin. Endocrinol. Metab.*, **70**, 403–9.

77 Mellinger, G.D., Balter, M.B., Uhlenhuth, E.H. (1985) Insomnia and its treatment. Prevalence and correlates. *Arch. Gen. Psychiatry*, **42**, 225–32.

78 Ford, D.E., Kamerow, D.B. (1989) Epidemiologic study of sleep disturbances and psychiatric disorders. An opportunity for prevention? *JAMA* **262**, 1479–84.

79 National Sleep Foundation. (1991) *Sleep in America: A National Survey of US Adults.* Princeton, NJ: Gallup Organization.

80 Lugaresi, E., Cirignotta, F., Coccagna, G., Piana, C. (1980) Some epidemiological data on snoring and cardiocirculatory disturbances. *Sleep*, **3**, 221–4.

81 Norton, P.G., Dunn, E.V. (1985) Snoring as a risk factor for disease: an epidemiological survey. *BMJ*, **291**, 630–2.

82 Young, T., Palta, M., Dempsey, J., Skatrud, J., Weber, S., Badr, S. (1993) The occurrence of sleep-disordered breathing among middle-aged adults. *N. Engl. J. Med.*, **328**, 1230–5.

83 Ohayon, M.M., Guilleminault, C., Priest, R.G., Caulet, M. (1997) Snoring and breathing pauses during sleep: telephone interview survey of a United Kingdom population sample. *BMJ*, **314**, 860–3.

84 Bearpark, H., Elliott, L., Grunstein, R., Cullen, S., Schneider, H., Althaus, W. *et al.* (1995) Snoring and sleep apnea. A population study in Australian men. *Am. J. Respir. Crit. Care Med.*, **151**, 1459–65.

85 Jennum, P., Sjol, A. (1992) Epidemiology of snoring and obstructive sleep apnoea in a Danish population, age 30–60. *J. Sleep Res.*, **1**, 240–4.

86 Namen, A.M., Wymer, A., Case, D., Haponik, E.F. (1999) Performance of sleep histories in an ambulatory medicine clinic: impact of simple chart reminders. *Chest*, **116**, 1558–63.

Obstructive sleep apnoea/hypopnoea syndrome

2

Introduction

Obstructive sleep apnoea/hypopnoea syndrome (OSAHS) is arguably the most prevalent disease to be discovered in the twentieth century. Unfortunately, its novelty means that many physicians graduated before sleep apnoea was included in the curriculum and some still have to increase their index of suspicion sufficiently to make the diagnosis appropriately. The consequences of missing the diagnosis can threaten the lives of sufferers and other road users. Further, the syndrome is one of the most satisfying conditions in medicine to treat, with major and rapid improvements in patients' quality of life, thus all physicians should be fully familiar with this common condition.

History

OSAHS is not a new condition, but a newly recognized one.[1,2] In the fourth century BC Dionysius, tyrant of Heraclea 'lived in fear of suffocation from fat, adopted a very curious mode of keeping himself awake'.[1] This consisted of having his attendants thrust needles through his sides into his belly to awaken him every time he fell asleep and this allowed him to breathe.

William Wadd was a surgeon who, in the early nineteenth century, described contemporary cases of sleepiness associated with obesity.[3] One man who weighed 23 stones (320 lbs, 145 kg) 'was withal so lethargic that he frequently fell asleep in company. He felt so much inconvenience and alarm . . . and was sent to Edinburgh to consult Dr Gregory' the Professor of Medicine. He was dieted successfully to 15 stones (210 lbs, 95 kg) and 'he is now well'.

The most famous nineteenth-century account of sleep apnoea was by Charles Dickens, in the *Pickwick Papers*, in the 1830s.[4] Dickens was in his twenties when he produced his remarkable description of Joe the fat boy, who was allegedly modelled on a James Budden who had bullied Dickens in his childhood. Joe weighed 280 lbs (130 kg) and was extraordinarily sleepy. On numerous occasions Pickwick utters in exasperation 'Joe – damn that boy, he's gone to sleep again'. He is reported to fall asleep during meals, after knocking on doors, during the firing of cannons and on a bed of stones. His snoring was loud and carried from 'the distant kitchen'. Joe suffered from the dropsy – right heart failure – and probably polycythaemia too as he was noted to be of ruddy complexion. All these features are now recognized to be hallmarks of end-stage sleep apnoea. However, the medical profession descriptions lagged behind Dickens.

In 1877, Dr William Broadbent, who later became an eminent London physician and was knighted, reported:[5]

> When a person . . . is lying on his back in heavy sleep and snoring loudly, it very commonly happens that every now and then the inspiration fails to overcome the resistance in the pharynx of which stertor or snoring is the audible sign, and there will be perfect silence through two, three or even four respiratory periods in which there are ineffectual chest movements; finally air enters with a loud snort . . .

Twelve years later, two English physicians reported further cases. Caton[6] reported to the Clinical Society of London a case of 'narcolepsy' in a 37-year-old man who had become sleepy in conjunction with weight gain:

> The moment he sat down sleep came on, and even when standing or walking . . . When in sound sleep a very peculiar state of the glottis is observed, a spasmodic closure entirely suspending respiration. The thorax and abdomen are seen to heave from fruitless contractions of inspiratory and expiratory muscles; their efforts increase in violence for about a minute to a minute and a half, the skin meantime becoming more and more cyanosed, until at last, when the condition to the onlooker is most alarming, the glottic obstruction yields . . .

The same year, Morison[7] reported a 63-year-old man with a 15-year history of increasing sleepiness, who would fall asleep playing cards and snore:

> I have myself observed him asleep in bed with an intensely cyanotic countenance, a condition from which he was roused after a snorting and choking sound had issued from his respiratory passages . . .

In 1937, Spitz, a German physician, described three patients who were sleepy, cyanosed and had right heart failure.[8] One of them had periodic breathing with apnoeas which were noted to end with a snore. The photographs of the patients showed the typical somnolence and large necks found in overweight patients with the sleep apnoea/hypopnoea syndrome. Weight loss was reported to reduce the sleepiness.

In 1956, Burwell reported a 51-year-old executive with a one-year history of somnolence associated with persistent and resistant ankle swelling. His admission to the Peter Bent Brigham Hospital appears to have been precipitated by annoyance at falling asleep when dealt a full house at poker and thus failing to capitalize on his luck![9] He weighed 263 lbs (120 kg) and had polycythaemia, right heart failure, hypoxaemia and hypercapnia and was noted to have apnoea. He lost 39 lbs (18 kg) and his sleepiness and 'periodic respiration' resolved. The similarity to Joe, Dickens' fat boy, was noted and the name 'Pickwickian syndrome' applied.

Jung and colleagues in Germany[10] and Gastaut and co-workers in France[11] simultaneously reported the recognition that the apnoeas caused the sleepiness in 1965. Both groups made recordings of sleep and breathing patterns in patients with the Pickwickian syndrome – obesity plus hypercapnic respiratory failure – and realized that the recurrent breathing pauses were associated with sleep disruption. Word spread throughout continental Europe and a French neurologist, Christian Guilleminault, played a major role in promoting the condition in North America.[12] The recognition by Colin Sullivan that continuous positive airway pressure (CPAP) would make an effective therapy represented a major advance.[13]

The medical profession in the UK was slow to recognize patients with the condition and, in 1981, a group of senior doctors interested in sleep wrote in the *Lancet* that the sleep apnoea syndrome 'was uncommon in Britain'.[14] However, this must have reflected a lack of clinical suspicion rather than absence of cases as patients began to be identified in the UK in the early 1980s and there has been an exponential growth in numbers since.

It became apparent that only a minority of end-stage patients had the polycythaemia and right heart failure typical of the Pickwickian syndrome, most having sleepiness plus apnoeas, and so the title 'sleep apnoea syndrome' was adopted.[12] Later, it was recognized that episodes where the breathing was reduced but did not stop – so-called hypopnoeas – could produce the same clinical picture[15] and the term 'obstructive sleep apnoea/hypopnoea syndrome' (OSAHS) emerged.

Definition of OSAHS

The definition has evolved over recent decades and will continue to evolve. A syndrome is the association of a clinical picture with specific abnormalities on investigation. The best current working definition is the co-existence of unexplained excessive daytime sleepiness or at least two other major symptoms with at least five obstructed breathing events per hour of sleep.[16] This threshold will probably need to be refined upwards and it will need to be clarified whether non-apnoeic non-hypopnoeic respiratory events are equally clinically relevant as apnoeas and hypopnoeas.

Apnoeas are defined in adults as a 10-second breathing pause[12] and hypopnoeas[15] as a 10-second event where there is continued breathing but the ventilation is reduced by at least 50 per cent from the previous baseline during sleep[16] (Figure 2.1).

Figure 2.1
Schematic of apnoeas and hypopnoeas. Apnoeas are 10-s cessations of airflow and hypopnoeas are 10-s periods when ventilation or thoraco-abdominal movement is reduced by at least 50 per cent.

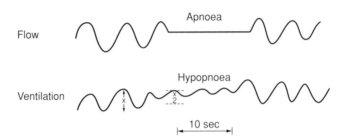

Another term used to describe recurrent episodes of airflow limitation during sleep without accompanying apnoeas is the upper airways resistance syndrome.[17,18] It is likely that this is part of the OSAHS spectrum and not a separate disease and is often identified due to technical limitations of methods used to detect hypopnoeas (*see* page 57). This is an area of considerable contention, however.[19]

Epidemiology

Although there have been a large number of studies of the prevalence of sleep apnoea/hypopnoea in the general population, few used ideal methods and it is difficult to draw firm conclusions. Broadly, the frequency of OSAHS – defined as the co-existence of sleepiness with irregular breathing at night – is in the range 0.3–4 per cent of the middle-aged male population[20–23] with most studies giving prevalences of 1–4 per cent.[21–23] The study giving the lowest prevalence[20] used oximetry alone and so may have underestimated the frequency of OSAHS, whereas those giving the highest prevalences may have overestimated obstructive events by including central apnoeas and breath holds occurring during wakefulness and respiratory events due to disturbed sleep resulting from the equipment/location.[21,22] Thus, a conservative estimate of prevalence of OSAHS in middle-aged men is 1–2 per cent. However, that is merely the prevalence of the association between sleepiness and irregular breathing during sleep, it is not an estimate of those who would benefit from diagnosis and treatment – that is not known. Nevertheless, 1–2 per cent makes OSAHS a common condition with a similar frequency to insulin-dependent diabetes or moderate or severe asthma in the middle-aged population.

The prevalence of OSAHS in middle-aged women has been less well studied but is probably about half that in men[21,23] at approximately 0.5–1 per cent.

The condition occurs in all ages, including children and the elderly, but data on prevalence outwith middle age are less clear. It has been suggested that OSAHS is slightly less common in the elderly than the middle-aged, but further work on this is needed. Certainly, the argument that the prevalence of OSAHS is lower in the elderly than in middle age because middle-aged OSAHS patients die of vascular disease is premature to say the least. The evidence is that irregular breathing during sleep is common in the elderly,[24] the difficulty may be that sleepiness becomes a more accepted symptom in this group.

There are relatively few data on the natural progression of OSAHS. In 55 untreated patients with moderate OSAHS, mean apnoea/hpopnoea index (AHI) increased from 22 to 33 in 18 months[25] and in 38 untreated subject AHI increased from four to 13 over 10 years.[26] In neither case was the increase associated with weight gain. However, a study of 32 patients over five years showed no change in apnoea plus hypopnoea frequency.[27]

Factors predisposing to apnoeas and hypopnoeas include age, male gender, obesity, smoking and alcohol consumption.[23] However, alcohol consumption in patients with OSAHS seems to be no different from that in the general population.[28]

Mechanism of upper airway narrowing

OSAHS results from narrowing of the upper airway during sleep. Despite some early suggestions that this might occur at laryngeal level, the site of narrowing is in the pharynx[29] (Figure 2.2).

In a pivotal study in 1978, Remmers and colleagues[29] not only demonstrated pharyngeal occlusion but showed that this was associated with decreased electromyographic tone in the genioglossal muscle of the tongue, and that pharyngeal reopening was co-incident with arousal and with reactivation of the genioglossus. These workers also noted that the airway occlusion was limited to inspiration and proposed the hypothesis that the negative pharyngeal pressure on inspiration sucked the airway closed when genioglossal tone was reduced during sleep.[29] This theory has been refined over the subsequent decades, but the principle that occlusion results from suction of the airway being inadequately opposed by upper airway dilating muscle

Figure 2.2
Schematic of the upper airway with the area of collapse during apnoeas and hypopnoeas shaded.

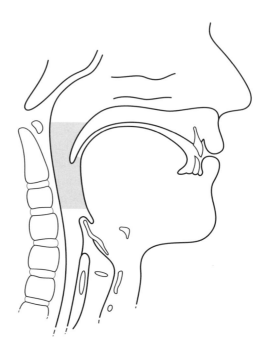

activity remains the cornerstone of our understanding of the syndrome. To appreciate the mechanism of upper airway obstruction it is first important to understand pharyngeal anatomy and function.

UPPER AIRWAY IN NORMAL SUBJECTS

The pharynx extends from the back of the nose to the larynx. It is a muscular tube which serves three purposes – respiration, swallowing and speech. Large tubes dedicated solely to respiration, such as the trachea, are semi-rigid and thus only mildly collapsible. Tubes solely for swallowing need to be able to have distensibility and co-ordinated peristalsis for bulk food propulsion, and speech requires fine adjustment of calibre and flow. Despite these three incompatible design needs, the pharynx fulfils these the roles satisfactorily during wakefulness, but not during sleep. The muscle hypotonia characteristic of sleep produces major respiratory problems because the pharynx becomes collapsible when intraluminal pressure falls in inspiration.

Upper airway muscles

Palate
The soft palate is a muscular structure comprising five different striated muscle groups (Figure 2.3). These are:

- **Palatoglossus** which forms the anterior tonsillar pillar. Its action is to move the palate downwards and forwards thus promoting nasal airflow, the normal route of breathing during sleep.
- **Palatopharyngeus** which forms the posterior tonsillar pillar and moves the palate downwards.
- **Levator palatini** which elevates the soft palate, promoting oral breathing.
- **Tensor palatini** which tightens the palate in the lateral plane and thus may contribute to rigidity.
- **Musculus uvulae** shortens the palate and may be involved in nasopharyngeal closure.

Most of these palatal muscles are true respiratory muscles, with obvious increases in electromyographic activity during inspiration in the palatoglossus,[30] the palatopharyngeus[31] and the levator palatini.[32] However, the tensor palatini shows no change in activity with the respiratory cycle[33] and it is unclear whether it really has a respiratory role. Nasal breathing is associated with increased activity of the palatoglossus[31] and palatopharyngeus[31] and decreased activity of levator palatini,[32] changes which are intuitively correct to promote nasal flow reinforcing the respiratory roles of these muscles. In addition, lying supine increases activity of the palatoglossus[30] and palatopharyngeus[31] during nasal breathing, again intuitively appropriate changes to promote nasal flow and counteract the effects of gravity on the soft palate and tongue.

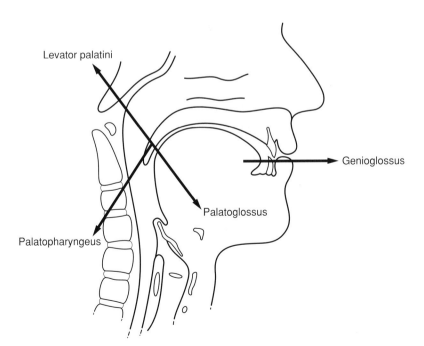

Figure 2.3
Direction of action of the upper airway muscles.

The tongue

The major tongue muscle, genioglossus, protrudes the tongue. The genioglossus tenses with each inspiration,[34] with nasal breathing.[35] Genioglossus also contracts on lying down[30,36] so increasing the retroglossal airway in supine awake normal subjects[37] or maintaining the retroglossal airway in supine awake patients with OSAHS.[38] Genioglossal strength declines with age.[39]

Hyoid muscles

The hyoid bone is attached directly or indirectly to the mandible by the mylohyoid and geniohyoid muscles. It also has inferior connections via the sternohyoid and omohyoid. The precise roles of these muscles in respiration in humans is unclear.

Reflex responses of upper airway muscles

Application of a negative pressure inside the pharynx results in rapid contraction of the genioglossus,[40] palatoglossus,[30] palatopharyngeus,[31] levator palatini[41] and tensor palatini.[42] The magnitude of the EMG response increases as more negative pressures are applied.[41] As all the main upper airway muscles react in the same way, it seems likely that this is a non-specific stiffening response to prevent upper airway collapse.

These responses are too rapid to be voluntary and must be reflex-driven.[43] The sensors for the reflex are in the upper airway[44] and the reflex may be blocked by a combination of local anaesthesia to the upper airway and superior laryngeal nerve block.[40] The sensors must be partly in the mucosa as local anaesthesia to the upper airway reduces but does not abolish the response,[30,45] raising the possibility that muscle spindles may also be involved.

Airway during wakefulness

In awake normal subjects pharyngeal size:

- Is greater in men than women in the seated position.[46,47]
- Is similar in men and women when supine.[47] This difference from the seated position probably reflects greater mass loading from increased neck muscle bulk and neck fat in men.[48]
- Decreases with obesity in men and women.[47]
- Diminishes with age in men[47,49] and women.[47]
- Increases with increasing lung volume.[50]

The male upper airway appears to be more compliant with greater changes in pharyngeal volume with lung volume[46] or posture changes.[47] Whether this is a real compliance difference or merely due to greater changes in airway length or mass loading in men remains to be proved.

Effects of sleep

Sleep generally produces hypotonia of striated muscle and the upper airway dilator muscles are not exceptions. The electromyographic tone of the palatoglossus[51] (Figure 2.4), levator palatini[51] and tensor palatini[33] have all been shown to decrease during non-REM sleep. One study has suggested that genioglossal EMG tone does not alter from wakefulness to non-REM sleep,[52] but it does decrease in eye-movement dense REM sleep in comparison to non-REM sleep.[53]

Sleep also has a marked effect on the response of the upper airways to negative pressure with delayed and decreased responses during non-REM sleep documented for the genioglossus[54] and tensor palatini[42] muscles. Adequate studies in REM sleep are awaited.

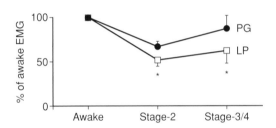

Figure 2.4
Decrease in muscle tone during non-REM sleep in palatoglossus (PG) and levator palatini (LP) muscles. (Adapted from Tangel et al.,[51] with permission.)

THE UPPER AIRWAY IN PATIENTS WITH OSAHS

Pharyngeal size in OSAHS patients awake

Patients with OSAHS have smaller upper airways than normal subjects when assessed in the supine position by computerized tomography (CT) scan[55,56] or resistance measurements[57] or when seated by acoustic reflection.[58,59] However, there is considerable overlap between the data points for normal subjects and patients OSAHS and none of these measurements are diagnostically useful. Patients with OSAHS have been reported to have upper airways which are more elliptical than those of normal subjects, with the long axis in the antero-posterior direction,[60,61] although this may be due to increased body mass and not specific to OSAHS.[62]

There are two main reasons for the differences in airway size between normal subjects and OSAHS patients – fat deposition and facial bone structure.

Effect of obesity

Obese patients with OSAHS have fat deposits lateral to the pharynx.[63-65] These are significantly larger than in weight-matched subjects without

OSAHS[63,64] but the differences are small amounting to less than 2 ml per subject.[64] Interestingly, non-obese OSAHS patients also have more fat deposited lateral to their upper airways than weight matched control subjects[65] (Figure 2.5), but again this is a small difference averaging only 3 ml. However, these observations in both obese and non-obese patients with OSAHS suggest that despite the small volume of fat involved, it may be important in the development of the condition. There is also considerably more adipose tissue in the subcutaneous tissues of OSAHS patients compared to weight-matched control subjects[65] and this may contribute to mass loading of the pharynx in patients when they lie down.

Facial structure

Retroposition of the maxilla and mandible predisposes to OSAHS,[66] by causing antero-posterior narrowing of the pharynx due to posterior displacement of the soft palate and tongue (Figure 2.6). These bony abnormalities are particularly common in non-obese OSAHS patients.[67] The structural changes are usually subtle and not seen on routine clinical inspection. However, either lateral cephalometry or orthodontic measurement[68] will detect them. These facial structural traits run in OSAHS families.[69]

There are many other differences between lateral cephalometry in normal subjects and patients with OSAHS, but most may be secondary to other changes. For example, while the enlarged soft palate observed in OSAHS patients may contribute to upper airway occlusion during sleep, it probably

Figure 2.5

Magnetic resonance imaging (MRI) of an OSAHS patient (A) and a weight-, age- and gender-matched healthy subject; (B) showing (1) the smaller upper airway in the OSAHS patient (black area in centre) and (2) the greater amount of adipose tissue in the OSAHS patient both lateral to the airway and in the subcutaneous tissues.

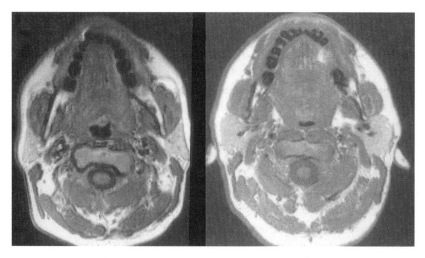

A   B

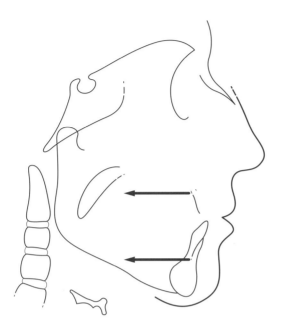

Figure 2.6
Facial structure in non-obese OSAHS patients with backward displacement of the maxilla and mandible resulting in upper airway narrowing.

results from local oedema caused by the trauma of snoring and airway occlusion,[70,71] and partly from muscle hypertrophy.[72] OSAHS patients may also have an increase in soft palatal fat which will primarily contribute to occlusion but there are no comparisons with weight-matched normal subjects.[72] Similarly, the inferior hyoid displacement found in obese OSAHS patients[73] may reflect fat deposition or age, and its pathogenic significance is questionable.

Combining facial structure and obesity

Overall, the risk of apnoeas and hypopnoeas during sleep seems largely to be related to, and predictable by, a combination of measurements of jaw shape and obesity.[62,68,74] Thinner SAHS patients are more likely to have shorter jaws and obese patients less likely to have craniofacial abnormalities.[67] Obese patients have narrower upper airways due to fat deposition, and weight loss results in less fat deposited around the upper airway and fewer apnoeas and hypopnoeas.[64]

Upper airway muscles in OSAHS

Patients with SAHS have increased palatal muscle bulk.[72] There is a change in muscle type in the genioglossus and palate of OSAHS patients with a shift towards those found with increased muscle use, more Type II A and less Type II B.[75] These muscles are also metabolically more active in OSAHS patients with increased levels of phosphorylase, phoshofructokinase, glyceraldehyde phosphate dehydrogenase and creatine kinase.[75] This alteration in muscle structure and function is believed to result from increased usage of these muscles to maintain airway patency. This increased use occurs both when awake[76] (Figure 2.7) and asleep.[77] The changes in genioglossal muscle reverse with CPAP therapy.[78]

The increased genioglossal activity when awake in patients with OSAHS compared to normal subjects[76] is to overcome the anatomical narrowing of the upper airway.[55,56] This is supported by recent data showing that weight loss in patients with OSAHS is associated with widening of the upper airway and decreased upper airway muscle activity during wakefulness.[79]

The upper airway muscles of patients with OSAHS, like those of normal subjects, respond to negative pressure.[41] However, when the response is assessed as a percentage rise of that individual's maximum EMG, the magnitude of the response is less in patients with OSAHS than in normal subjects[41] (Figure 2.8). As the force generation of palatal muscles cannot currently be measured *in vivo*, it is impossible to determine whether this difference in percentage maximal response reflects increased muscle strength in OSAHS patients – and thus perhaps negative pressure could result in similar force generation at a lower percentage maximum EMG – or to a genuine difference in reflex sensitivity. Patients re-studied after CPAP therapy had a significant improvement in their EMG response to negative pressure, and this change was apparent within two weeks of starting CPAP[41], too soon for muscle atrophy to occur, suggesting reflex sub-sensitivity in untreated OSAHS.

There is histological evidence of sensory neuropathic changes in the palate of OSAHS patients perhaps produced by vibration[80] and this could con-

Figure 2.7

Peak genioglossal EMG during wakefulness is higher in OSAHS patients than normal control subjects *$P<0.05$ vs controls. (Adapted from Mezzanotte et al.,[76] with permission.)

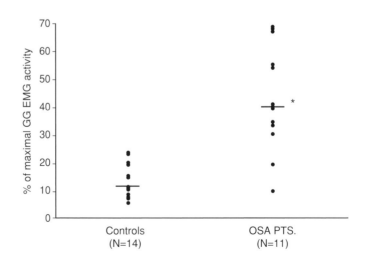

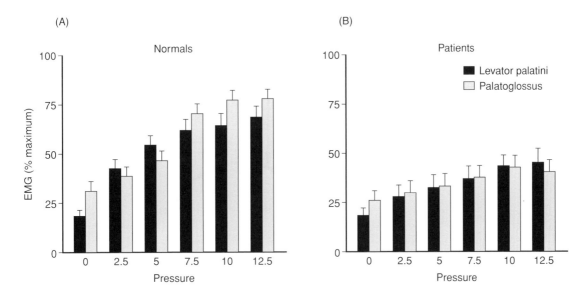

(A) Normals

(B) Patients

Levator palatini
Palatoglossus

Figure 2.8
Responses of levator palatini (solid) and palatoglossus (hatched) muscles to negative upper airway pressure in (A) normal subjects and (B) OSAHS patients, showing the lower responses in the patients. (Adapted from Mortimore and Douglas,[41] with permission.)

tribute to decreased sensitivity to negative pressure. Another possible explanation is mucosal oedema from airway trauma which reverses with CPAP therapy.[71]

Upper airway during sleep in patients with OSAHS

Obstructive apnoeas and hypopnoeas during sleep are caused by occlusion or narrowing of the pharyngeal airway.[29] The factors predisposing to occlusion include obesity and facial structure with the addition of sleep state related changes in upper airway dilator muscle tone (Figure 2.9).

There have been relatively few recordings of upper airway muscle activity during obstructive apnoeas. These have shown decreased dilator muscle activity during apnoeas[46] with no change in constrictor muscle activity. Towards the end of apnoeas and hypopnoeas, upper airway dilator muscle activity increases, rising further with the arousal[77] (Figure 2.10) which terminates the event.

Such apnoeas and hypopnoeas are most common in light sleep (stages 1 and 2) and REM sleep and relatively unusual during slow wave sleep (stages 3 and 4).[81] This is compatible with evidence that the upper airway is less collapsible during slow wave than in the other sleep stages.[82]

An index of upper airway collapsibility may be obtained by artificially varying the pressure in a nasal mask in a sleeping subject and plotting the relationship between nasal pressure and inspiratory flow. The nasal pressure at which the extrapolated flow reaches zero is the critical closing pressure, or Pcrit. During non-REM sleep, Pcrit is negative in normal subjects, positive

Figure 2.9
Factors predisposing to upper airway occlusion in OSAHS.

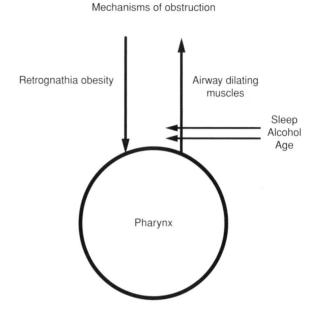

Figure 2.10
Genioglossal tone in the three breaths before, and the first three inspiratory attempts after apnoeas, followed by the last three efforts of the apnoeas and first three post-apnoeic breaths. Data (adapted from Surratt et al.,[77] with permission) shows the decline in genioglossal tone immediately before and during apnoeas, rising with arousal at apnoea termination.

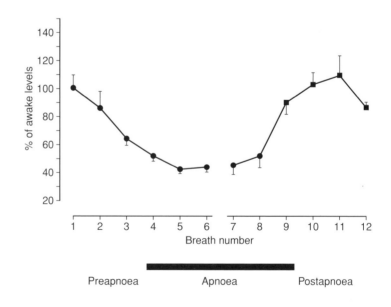

in patients with OSAHS and intermediate in snorers.[83] Pcrit decreases – and thus upper airway collapsibility decreases – with weight loss in OSAHS patients.[84] Pcrit increases – and thus collapsibility increases – with sleep fragmentation[85] and with mouth opening during sleep.[86] Endoscopic visualization has showed that the upper airway occluded at positive pressures in 85 per cent of OSAHS patients.[87]

Site of obstruction

Studies using either endoscopic or manometric methods to determine the precise location of maximal narrowing or occlusion in the pharynx in sleeping patients with OSAHS have shown that it varies between patients. In approximately half, narrowing is greatest in the retro-palatal area and half retro-glossally.[88,89] However, in all patients there is generalized narrowing of the pharynx and the precise point of first occlusion or maximal narrowing may be of academic rather than pathophysiological or therapeutic importance.[90]

Arousal response

Patients with the sleep apnoea/hypopnoea syndrome are not awoken purely by hypoxaemia.[91] Nor, in isolation, does the resulting minor hypercapnia[92] nor increased airflow resistance[93] produce awakenings. Patients tend to arouse at a specific level of pleural pressure[94] once sufficient respiratory effort has been stimulated. It is not clear whether the sensor for the arousal response to the intrathoracic pressure is in the chest wall or lungs. Interestingly, normal subjects exposed to hypoxia, hypercapnia or increased airflow resistance also waken at the same level of pleural pressure independent of the stimulus used.[93]

CONSEQUENCES OF AROUSAL

Arousal from sleep results in two distinct consequences[95] (Figure 2.11). First, there is the obvious sequel of sleep disruption, which contribute as to the daytime consequences of sleepiness and impaired cognitive performance.[96] Second, arousal is associated with autonomic changes including elevation of arterial blood pressure[97] which may contribute to increased cardiovascular and cerebrovascular risk in patients with OSAHS.

Daytime function in OSAHS

Patients with OSAHS are usually sleepy and often report concentration difficulties. Psychometric testing demonstrates impaired cognitive perfor-

Figure 2.11

Effect of sleep disruption on patients with OSAHS.

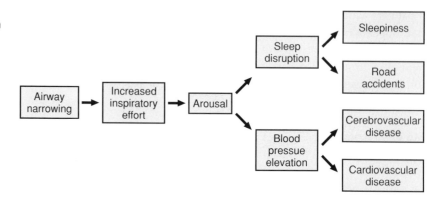

mance.[96] These changes are, at least in part, caused by the recurrent arousals from sleep as disturbing a single night's sleep with sound-induced arousals every two minutes produces similar sleepiness and defects in daytime function.[98] However, there may also be contributions from the hypoxaemia associated with the apnoeas and hypopnoeas as the extent of nocturnal hypoxaemia correlates better with daytime function changes than the frequency of EEG arousals.[99,100] One study has suggested that the daytime function deficits in patients with OSAHS correlate best with more sophisticated measures of arousal, such as alterations in pulse transit time or neural net analysis of the EEG.[101] This is compatible with evidence that sleepiness and impaired cognitive function can be produced by sound-induced arousals from sleep which were too minor to be detected by standard EEG criteria.[102]

One of the problems with many of these studies in OSAHS is that they examine correlations in daytime function across populations of OSAHS patients and cannot allow for the large pre-morbid differences in education, intelligence, age, sleep ability or other factors. Recent studies of patients' function before and after successful treatment indicate poor correlations between arousal frequency measured by conventional ASDA criteria and improvement in objective outcomes.[103,100]

Blood pressure at arousal

Arousal from sleep causes a rise in arterial blood pressure, irrespective of the cause of arousal. Thus wakenings due to noise,[98] apnoeas and hypopnoeas[97] (Figure 2.12) and leg jerks[104] are all associated with a blood pressure rise. During sleep, blood pressure is normally lower than during wakefulness[105,106] and the post-arousal blood pressure may be markedly higher than the patient's usual waking pressure. Thus OSAHS patients with recurrent arousals may have a resulting increase in their cardiovas-

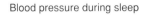

Blood pressure during sleep

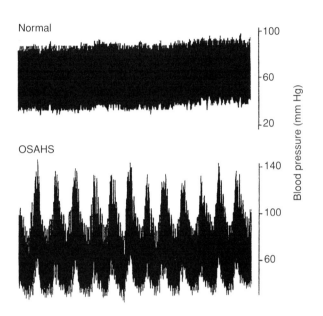

Figure 2.12
Beat-by-beat blood
pressure during sleep in a
normal subject and in an
OSAHS patient with
recurrent arousals.
(Adapted from Davies *et al.*,
(1994) Non-invasive beat
to beat arterial blood
pressure during non-REM
sleep in obstructive sleep
apnoea and snoring.
Thorax, 49, 335–9, with
permission from the BMJ
Publishing Group.)

cular load each night, which over years may become clinically significant (*see* page 42).

Distribution of apnoeas and hypopnoeas during the night

Apnoeas and hypopnoeas are usually more common and last longer in stages 1 and 2 rather than stages 3 and 4 sleep, and most common and longest in REM sleep.[81] Some patients have apnoeas and hypopnoeas in REM sleep only and this has been termed 'REM-related OSAHS'. Apnoeas and hypopnoeas tend to become slightly more prolonged later in the night.[107] The reason for this is unclear but may relate to progressive blunting of arousal response by sleep fragmentation.

In patients with mild-to-moderate OSAHS, apnoeas and hypopnoeas are more common in the supine than in lateral lying positions, and some patients have exclusively posturally related OSAHS with events when supine only.[108] Some patients with severe OSAHS find they sleep better sitting than lying and have adopted this habit, which minimizes apnoeas and hypopnoeas, before seeking medical help.

Genetics

Snoring runs in families and so several studies have investigated whether sleep apnoea/hypopnoea is also familial. There is now firm evidence that OSAHS is more common in the family members of OSAHS sufferers than in the general population[69,109] (Figure 2.13), and that this relationship is independent of the well-known familial nature of obesity.[110] The precise mechanism of this association awaits further research, but it partly relates – at least in thinner patients – to familial facial structure with back-setting of the jaw[69] (*see* Figure 2.6). Other factors under investigation include genetically determined differences in selective deposition of adipose tissue around the upper airway, upper airway dilator muscle function, ventilatory control and susceptibility to sleepiness.

Figure 2.13
Apnoea plus hypopnoea frequency is higher in relatives of non-obese OSAHS patients in comparison to age-, gender-, height- and weight-matched normal subjects. (Adapted from Mathur and Douglas,[69] with permission.)

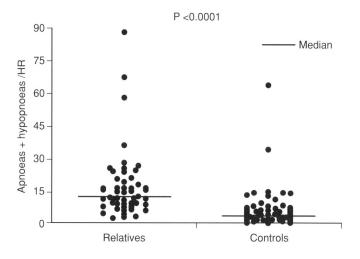

Complications and associations of OSAHS

ACCIDENTS

Many patients will admit to falling asleep at the wheel and over a third to having had an accident or nearly had an accident because of falling asleep when driving.[111] This has to be set in the context that falling asleep at the wheel is not uncommon in the general population, with 19 per cent of men admitting to falling asleep driving[112] and 29 per cent close to doing so in the past year.[112,113] Nevertheless, sleepiness at the wheel is a recurrent problem for many OSAHS patients but an exceptional occurrence in the normal population, when it is usually associated with acute sleep deprivation, overnight driving or shift working. Under-reporting of sleep-related driving problems by OSAHS patients is common.[111]

As well as self-reported driving difficulties, there is clear objective evidence of a 1.3–12-fold increase in accident rates among those with sleep apnoea.[114–119] These studies have been carried out using a variety of approaches. Prospectively gathered accident rates in OSAHS patients have been found to be 1.3–7-fold higher than those in the general population.[117–119] Epidemiological studies comparing accident rates in individuals from the general population found a seven-fold increased risk of having had multiple road accidents in those with more than 15 apnoeas plus hypopnoeas per hour of sleep in comparison to non-snoring normal subjects.[115] A Spanish study in which drivers involved in road accidents were compared with control subjects found that those with more than 10 apnoeas plus hypopnoeas per hour of sleep were six times more likely to be drivers involved in road accidents than those without sleep apnoea.[114]

There is also convincing evidence from vigilance tasks and driving simulators[120–122] that driving performance is impaired in patients with OSAHS. Indeed, drunk normal subjects perform better on a driving simulator than sober OSAHS patients[123] (Figure 2.14). Interestingly, the impairment is not just limited to periods when patients actually fall asleep; their response is also impaired when they are awake, due to impaired vigilance[124] and delayed reaction times. CPAP improves performance on vigilance and driving simulator tasks.[120,125,126] The link between OSAHS and accidents is further proved by evidence that the road accident rate in OSAHS is reduced by 40 per cent by treatment with CPAP.[127,128]

Little attention has been paid to accidents at work, but there is some evidence that OSAHS patients have a 50 per cent increased risk of work place accidents.[129]

NEUROPSYCHOLOGICAL IMPAIRMENT

There have been relatively few good-quality studies examining neuropsychological function in OSAHS patients in comparison to an adequate number of well-matched control subjects, and indeed, because of the wide range of abilities in the community such studies are very difficult to perform. However, some[130,131] also and correlational[115,132] studies have suggested that cognitive function is impaired in OSAHS patients.[96] More convincingly, studies have shown marked improvements after CPAP treatment,[133–135] indicating that cognition was impaired by OSAHS. The deficits are broad rang-

Figure 2.14
Steering error on a driving simulator in OSAHS patients and control subjects matched for gender and driving experience. The control subjects were studied both sober and with a mean blood alcohol of 95 mg per cent. The sober OSAHS patients drove worse than the drunk (or sober) normal subjects. (Adapted from George et al.,[123] with permission.)

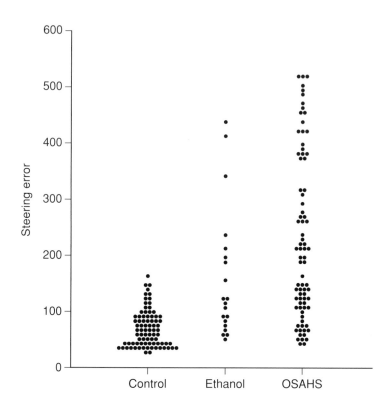

ing affecting attention, concentration, vigilance, manual dexterity, visuomotor skills, memory, verbal fluency and executive function.[96]

HYPERTENSION

Early epidemiological investigations showed an increase in hypertension among snorers,[136,137] but confounding factors, such as obesity, age, gender and alcohol consumption, make interpretation of these observations difficult.[138] Several studies also suggested an increase in hypertension in patients with OSAHS[139–141] and an increased frequency of OSAHS in patients with hypertension,[142–144] but most had similar problems with confounders.

Studies in an elegant computerized dog model[145] demonstrated that recurrent apnoeas produce both recurrent blood pressure rises from sleep and sustained daytime hypertension. However, while both apnoeas and recurrent arousals produce recurrent rises in blood pressure during the night, recurrent arousal without apnoea does not influence daytime blood pressure.[146] This suggests that the combination of arousal with some consequence of obstructive apnoea – either hypoxaemia or changes in intrathoracic pressure – are needed to affect daytime blood pressure. Studies in rats suggest that intermittent nocturnal hypoxaemia on its own can produce daytime hypertension even in the absence of upper airway obstruction.[147,148] Recurrent acoustic arousals produced synchronous transient hypertension but not sustained daytime hypertension in rats.[149]

Recent epidemiological studies in normal populations in which strenuous attempts have been made to exclude the effect of confounders strongly suggest an association between apnoeic activity during sleep and daytime hypertension.[150–152] Convincing evidence comes from the Wisconsin cohort study in which 1060 members of the working population had their breathing studied during sleep and then were followed up. At the original investigation, those found to have more than 25 apnoeas plus hypopnoeas per hour of sleep had a five-fold risk of being hypertensive.[150] The increase in risk of hypertension was greater in thinner patients who had abnormal breathing during sleep.[153] After four years, those with more than 15 apnoeas had a 2.9-fold increased chance of developing new hypertension[151] independent of confounders. Other cross-sectional studies in normal populations[152,154] or in OSAHS patients[155–157] have also indicated a 1.4–7-fold increased risk of hypertension once allowance has been made for other risk factors.

A carefully conducted case-control study found that patients with OSAHS had significantly higher blood pressures than matched control subjects, but that these increases were only significant during the sleeping period and in the afternoon.[158] Further and direct evidence that OSAHS causes hypertension comes from a study showing that CPAP therapy reduces 24-hour diastolic blood pressure[159] but the overall decrease was small, averaging 1.5 mm Hg over the 24 hours ($p<0.04$) and the decrease was only significant between the hours of 2 a.m. and 10 a.m. The decrease was greater in those with significant nocturnal hypoxaemia with more than 20 four per cent desaturations per hour of sleep, in whom the mean 24-hour diastolic blood pressure fall was 5 mm Hg.

Taken together, these studies convincingly indicate that OSAHS causes elevation of systemic blood pressure which is most marked during the hours of sleep. Averaged over the 24-hour day, this increase may be relatively small but it must be seen in the context that a 5 mm Hg fall in 24-hour diastolic pressure decreases cardiac risk by 20 per cent and stroke risk by 40 per cent over a 5–10-year period.[160,161]

MYOCARDIAL INFARCTION

There is no convincing evidence of an association between OSAHS and cardiac disease. One study has shown a slight increase in the frequency of apnoeas in patients who have had myocardial infarctions compared to control subjects.[162] However, although the difference was statistically significant, it was numerically small – mean 6.9 versus 1.4 apnoeas per hour – and of dubious clinical significance. Further, the apnoeas could have resulted from, rather than caused, the myocardial infarctions as cardiac failure is associated with Cheyne–Stokes respiration and central apnoeas during sleep.[163]

Other studies have suggested an excess of vascular deaths in patients with OSAHS,[164,165] but this does not prove causality as there are so many common risk factors for both conditions, including obesity, middle age and male gender. The American Sleep Heart Health Study found a 1.3-fold (95 per cent confidence interval 1.0–1.7) increased frequency of self-reported cardiovascular disease in those in the highest quartile of apnoea/hypopnoea frequency in comparison to the lowest quartile once allowance had been made for co-morbidities including age, gender, smoking, obesity, hypertension and diabetes.[166] Given the firm association between OSAHS and hypertension, it seems inevitable that OSAHS does predispose to ischaemic heart disease, but the current data is inadequate to be categorical.

STROKE

Similarly, there is insufficient evidence that OSAHS causes strokes. Irregular breathing during sleep is very common after strokes[167–169] but there is debate whether this is a consequence or cause of stroke. As yet there are no long-term studies showing a higher risk of stroke in individuals with disturbed breathing during sleep. Several studies do suggest that snoring is associated with an increased frequency of stroke.[170–173] Although some of these studies have relied on patients' recall of snoring and thus may be criticized for possible ascertainment bias,[172,173] longitudinal studies of populations whose snoring history was recorded at baseline have also shown an increased frequency of stroke in snorers.[170] However, the overlap of risk factors makes it impossible to conclude that upper airway narrowing during sleep causes stroke.

Stroke may cause Cheyne–Stokes respiration with recurrent central apnoeas, but obstructive events are also common. The high frequency of apnoeas and hypopnoeas during sleep in patients who have had strokes raises the question whether treatment of these events would help either their functional recovery or the prevention of recurrence of their stroke. Neither question has yet been answered.

RIGHT HEART FAILURE

Cardiac failure can be both caused by and cause apnoeas and hypopnoeas during sleep. Cheyne–Stokes breathing with central apnoeas can result from heart failure[163] and is discussed on page 233. Right heart failure can result from OSAHS,[9] and this was the original Pickwickian syndrome. Right heart failure occurs especially if the patient has daytime hypoxaemia as a consequence of co-existing lung or restrictive chest wall disease.[174,175] Most such patients will have chronic obstructive pulmonary disease, but some will have gross obesity impairing chest movement and a few will have neuromuscular diseases affecting the chest wall. Such patients then have two causes of sleep-related hypoxaemia and become more severely hypoxaemic during sleep than do other OSAHS patients. The hypoxaemia produces pulmonary hypertension and thus right heart failure may eventually ensue.

RESPIRATORY FAILURE

OSAHS patients with co-existing lung disease are more likely to develop daytime hypoxaemia and hypercapnia than others.[176] Usually the lung disease is chronic obstructive pulmonary disease (COPD). The ventilatory failure responds to treatment of the OSAHS[177] which is accompanied by recovery of respiratory drive.[178]

POLYCYTHAEMIA

Similarly, patients with both OSAHS and a co-existing condition causing daytime hypoxaemia may develop secondary polycythaemia. However, this is rare and there is as yet no evidence that patients with OSAHS have increased erythropoeitin levels.[179,180] Treatment should be directed at the OSAHS and the respiratory condition rather than at the polycythaemia.

ANAESTHETIC RISK

Patients with OSAHS are at increased risk peri-operatively as their upper airway may obstruct during the recovery period or as a consequence of sedation. Patients who anaesthetists have difficulty intubating are much more likely to have irregular breathing during sleep, with eight of 15 difficult-to-intubate patients having an AHI greater than 10 in comparison to two of 15 control subjects.[181] Anaesthetists should thus take sleep histories on all patients pre-operatively and take the appropriate precautions with those who might have OSAHS. This should include referring all those suspected of having OSAHS for investigation and in some situations operations may need to be delayed until the OSAHS is treated.

SUDDEN INFANT DEATH SYNDROME

There is debate whether there is an association between OSAHS and sudden infant death syndrome (SIDS). There is some evidence of a possible association, including the observation of a small increase in the frequency of obstructive apnoeas during sleep in infants who subsequently die from SIDS,[182] and an increased reporting of possible SIDS cases in families of patients with OSAHS.[183,184] There is also evidence of narrower upper airways in SIDS victims[185] and back-setting of the maxilla both in SIDS victims[186] and in the families with OSAHS reporting possible SIDS cases.[183]

Although it is possible that some cases of SIDS might be due to upper airway occlusion during sleep in association with immaturity in the arousal response resulting in failure to reopen the airway, this is far from proven. Patients with OSAHS who are potential or new parents should be reassured that there is no clear link and advised to take the normal precautions to avoid SIDS, including putting babies to sleep on their back, avoiding overheating them and banning smoking in the house.

Clinical features

SYMPTOMS

The dominant symptoms of OSAHS are sleepiness and difficulty concentrating[16,187] (Table 2.1).

Table 2.1
Symptoms of OSAHS

Sleepiness
Difficulty concentrating
Daytime fatigue
Unrefreshing sleep
Nocturnal choking
Nocturia
Depression
Decreased libido
Partner's report:
Snoring
Apnoeas
Restless sleep
Irritability

Sleepiness

Over 90 per cent of patients report sleepiness. This is not an invariable finding, perhaps because some patients have lost their frame of reference for 'normal' sleepiness. Alternatively, some may present early, aware that their ability to concentrate is impaired but before they become excessively sleepy. Also, those working on their feet may have no opportunity to be sleepy at work although they will usually report sleepiness after work.

Indeed, there is no gold standard definition of pathological subjective sleepiness. It is important to note whether the patient falls asleep frequently against his or her will, and particularly whether this occurs in dangerous situations, such as when driving. Various scales which have been developed to quantify sleepiness are often poorly related to either the severity of objective sleepiness or to the severity of SAHS.

The most widely used scale, the Epworth sleepiness scale (ESS) drawn up by Johns and named after the Melbourne district of its origin,[188] asks patients to rate their likelihood of falling asleep in eight different situations (Table 2.2). The original report by Johns[188] suggested that an ESS score of over 10/24 was abnormal. A larger study using a British normal population of middle-aged people suggested that the 95th percentile for ESS was 11.[189] Thus I regard an ESS score of 12/24 or more as abnormally sleepy.

Table 2.2
Epworth sleepiness scale

How often are you likely to doze off or fall asleep in the following situations, in contrast to feeling just tired? This refers to your usual way of life in recent times. Even if you have not done some of these things recently try to work out how they would have affected you. Use the following scale to choose the *most appropriate number* for each situation:

    0 = would *never* doze
    1 = *slight* chance of dozing
    2 = *moderate* chance of dozing
    3 = *high* chance of dozing

Situation	Chance of dozing
Sitting and reading	....
Watching TV	....
Sitting, inactive in a public place (e.g. theatre or a meeting)	....
As a passenger in a car for an hour without a break	....
Lying down to rest in the afternoon when circumstances permit	....
Sitting and talking to someone	....
Sitting quietly after lunch without alcohol	....
In a car, while stopped for a few minutes in traffic	....

Total ex 24 _____

Unfortunately, the correlation between ESS score and OSAHS severity is not good.[99] This is equally true whether the patient's or their partner's estimation of ESS is used.[190] Part of this may be due to perception problems as the patient's perception of his sleepiness is sharper after his OSAHS is treated; patients on treatment consistently scoring themselves as having been more sleepy prior to treatment than they originally reported at presentation.[111]

In practice, the Epworth score can be a clinically useful pointer to whether patients perceives themselves to have a problem with falling asleep. A high score should alert the clinician to the need to find a cause (*see* Chapter 5). An ESS score of <12, if corroborated by the partner and also by direct questioning showing no problems falling asleep driving or against the patient's will, suggests that sleepiness is not a clinical problem. However, as with any other self- or partner-reported symptom, there are exceptions. Those whose livelihoods depend on continuing to drive, fly or operate other dangerous machinery may perceive gain from under-reporting their sleepiness and often their partner shares these concerns.

Sleepiness is particularly a problem in monotonous situations such as watching television or films, listening to lectures or concerts or working for long periods with computers. Such sleepiness can have a major effect on the ability to work. We have patients who have slept whilst chairing board meetings, delivering lectures and sermons and examining patients as well as large numbers who have slept in less stimulating situations, such as on production lines and while working as security guards. Falling asleep in company, particularly in the evening is common and often has a markedly deleterious effect on the patient's – and their partner's – social life especially when it is recurrent and the slumber is punctuated by loud snoring.

Unfortunately, driving can also be boring, and many patients report difficulty with sleepiness particularly on long drives on major highways. Many report having to pull off the road on numerous occasions for a nap, and most will have developed strategies for dealing with sleepiness driving, usually opening windows, cooling the car and turning up their music. However, some strategies are bizarre such as a patient of mine who judged how sleepy he was by how often he had to stop the car to refill the water-pistol which his son used to squirt him anytime he appeared to be nodding off! Some will only drive if they have a partner with them to take over when they get sleepy. Many will have limited their driving to short distances for fear of falling asleep at the wheel. We also have patients who admit to falling asleep while driving buses, trucks and trains and when flying a light aircraft.

Impaired concentration

Some patients will absolutely deny any problems with sleepiness but may be seriously inconvenienced by difficulty concentrating and impaired work performance. They are usually aware that they are more mentally tired than before but see themselves at no risk of falling asleep. Impaired concentration may thus be a very difficult symptom to assess. Depression, anxiety and dementia often enter the differential diagnosis. Nevertheless, poor concentration is often a dominant feature in sleep apnoea and whenever it is associated with other pointers to the syndrome the patient should be investigated for OSAHS. The situation is further confused as depression is a common sequel of OSAHS.[96,191]

Unrefreshing sleep

Most OSAHS patients report that their sleep is unrefreshing. After a normal duration of nocturnal sleep they waken feeling still sleepy. The majority believe they sleep fairly soundly and are unaware of the recurrent arousals from sleep which are too brief to be recalled.

Nocturnal choking

Around a third of patients[187] recall waking up choking intermittently and some describe vividly episodes where they awaken but are unable to breath for many seconds. Some patients have run from the house to their garden in understandable panic before being able to breathe. Such episode seem to be more common in patients with only a few apnoeas and hypopnoeas per night, giving the impression that the cortical arousal response is blunted in more severe OSAHS. Nocturnal choking attacks need to be differentiated from left heart failure and nocturnal asthma, usually easy on the basis of the attacks lasting seconds with total resolution instantly thereafter, their occurrence around sleep onset as a rule and the association with loud snoring.

Other symptoms

Another sleep-related symptom of OSAHS is nocturia. This is associated with increased salt and water excretion during the night, and disappears with treatment of OSAHS.[192] The mechanism is believed to be increased atrial filling during the negative pressure swings of the obstructive events causing increased atrial natriuretic peptide secretion.[193]

Decreased libido is reported by many patients,[187] particularly the younger ones.

Morning headache was initially reported to be a feature of OSAHS, but whether this is a true association is debatable.[194] There is no doubt that patients with respiratory failure who hypoventilate during sleep may have morning headaches due to CO_2 retention[195] but the evidence for this in uncomplicated OSAHS is not compelling.

Weight gain

Patients should be asked about the relationship of developing symptoms to any weight gain. This may be therapeutically useful information as the presence of severe symptoms before weight gain will indicate that diet alone will not suffice.

Nasal symptoms

Problems with the nose and sinus should be documented, again for consideration when treatment is being planned. Any increase in nasal resistance will make inspiratory pressures more negative and predispose to upper airway obstruction.

Depression

Many OSAHS patients report feeling depressed and this improves with effective therapy.[191] As depression itself may cause sleepiness, it can be difficult to determine on history alone whether the sleepiness and depression are both caused by OSAHS or whether the patient is a simple snorer with depression.

PARTNER'S REPORT

OSAHS affects both sufferers and their families, particularly partners. The bed-partner is the best witness to what happens during the night and also can provide a useful independent check on the presence and severity of sleepiness. Thus, if possible, a history should always be obtained from the patient's partner. We send questionnaires to all partners – as well as to all patients – before their first consultation to ensure having the partner's story, even if he or she is unable to attend the consultation.

Snoring

Almost all partners of OSAHS patients will report loud snoring – 96 per cent in one series.[187] The few patients without a history of snoring may have never had a partner or witness or have a deaf or somnolent partner. A very few patients with OSAHS have an alert partner with good hearing who absolutely deny that their partner ever snored.[187] Snoring usually occurs every night and in severe OSAHS happens in all body postures. The volume of the snoring can match that of pneumatic drills or motorbikes. Partners and work-mates often initiate referral for treatment because of the unbearable noise. We have had patients referred because of pressure from family members unable to escape the noise anywhere in the house, from neighbours and from passers-by on the street!

The noise of the snoring can be a major problem for all concerned, not only for the family members. Vacations may be planned to avoid staying with friends lest they are disturbed, and hotels may be chosen to optimize soundproofing. Business trips may be highly embarrassing if shared rooms cannot be avoided. Working off-shore or at sea can also be difficult.

Apnoeas

Most partners will have noticed breathing pauses and for many these are the prime concern. Some will have timed their duration and frequency, others come armed with video recordings. Some partners will not have noticed frank breathing pauses but will have found that the snoring has the characteristic gaps. Indeed, the presence of loud but intermittent snoring is one of the best pointers to the occurrence of OSAHS.[196–198]

Restless sleep

Many partners will complain that the patient thrashes around in bed at night. This is apnoea-related. These movements not only disturb their partners sleep but may also be a major cause for strife, resulting in an underslept partner and sometimes in physical injury, particularly when the restless patient is large and flailing limbs strike the partner.

Irritability

Most partners of OSAHS patients report the patient is much more irritable than before. This often harms family life.

EXAMINATION

Physical examination is not as vital as history in making the diagnosis of OSAHS, but it is critical to the exclusion of other causes for the patient's symptoms and to the detection of causes and consequences of OSAHS and thus to the planning of treatment. The key factors to be noted include the following.

Obesity

Approximately 50 per cent of patients with the OSAHS are technically obese – that is, their body mass index [BMI; weight in kg/(height in metres)^2] is above 30 kg/m^2. It is important to ensure that height and weight are documented at first visit, and weight at all follow-up visits.

Neck circumference is better than BMI for predicting the likelihood of having OSAHS.[20,199] However, the improvement in predictive power is relatively small and I do not routinely measure neck size but note BMI and whether clinically the patient has a 'bull' neck.

Jaw structure

Backset jaws predispose to OSAHS.[66,67] Although visual inspection is not a sensitive way to detect minor degrees of retrognathia, this is a useful first step and will detect gross examples in patients who might benefit from corrective surgery.

Mouth

Tongue size should be assessed as macroglossia is common in sleep apnoea. This is best done by noting whether the tongue crowds the mouth, rising above the lower teeth and obscures the view of the uvula. The extent of the patient's own dentition should be noted as this may determine the applicability and type of oral appliance that can be used for treatment.

Pharynx

Tonsillar enlargement should be sought. A large red and oedematous uvula is normal in OSAHS and the throat is often narrowed in either the antero-posterior or lateral dimension.[200] Very rarely a lesion of the tongue or upper airway – such as a haemangioma – may be seen, which can be usefully corrected.

Nose

A gross inspection of nasal patency should be made in all patients. Those with problems should be referred for a specialist ENT opinion (*see* page 74).

Cardiovascular system

Blood pressure must be measured and an appropriate-sized cuff used to prevent the overestimation of pressure by use of a standard cuff on an over-sized arm. Ankle oedema and right ventricular heave should be sought specifically.

Respiratory system

Physicians should seek evidence of co-existing lung disease or chest wall disease, as patients with the combination of OSAHS with these conditions are more likely to have right heart failure[174] and ventilatory failure.[176] Ventilatory failure and ventilatory response may improve when OSAHS is treated.[201]

Neurological examination

Features of myotonic dystrophy or other neurological conditions associated with OSAHS should be considered in all patients.

Signs of predisposing conditions

The possibility of hypothyroidism,[202] acromegaly[156] and Marfan's syndrome[203] as causes for OSAHS should always considered.

Diagnosing OSAHS

INDEX OF SUSPICION

One of the biggest hurdles in making the diagnosis of OSAHS is that many doctors do not consider the possibility unless patients present with sleepiness plus snoring as their prime complaints. It is important to remember that patients with OSAHS often complain about their non-specific symptoms, such as difficulties with concentration, work or family problems and depression. Thus a high index of suspicion is needed to make the diagnosis in such patients. Sleep histories should be part of routine clinical practice.

DIFFERENTIAL DIAGNOSIS

Alternative causes of sleepiness are discussed over the next three chapters and in detail in Chapter 5. However, the main differential diagnoses which need to be considered are listed in Table 2.3.

Inadequate sleep
Shift work
Depression
Drugs
Narcolepsy
Idiopathic hypersomnolence
Restless leg syndrome/periodic limb movement disorder
Sleep phase disorders

Table 2.3
Other causes of sleepiness to be considered in possible OSAHS

PREDICTION EQUATIONS

Various equations have been developed to help predict the likelihood of a patient having the sleep apnoea/hypopnoea syndrom from historical and physical features.[68,196–198,204,205] In routine clinical practice these are not cost-effective. In our practice the following questions are asked:

1   Does this patient need to be investigated for possible OSAHS?

The answer is yes if patients – or their partners say they are: falling asleep regularly against their will; often sleepy when driving; not sleepy but complaining of at least two other major symptoms of OSAHS; contemplating surgery for snoring.

2   Should this patient be prioritized for an urgent sleep study?

The answer is yes if patients – or their partners say they are – at risk when driving; having major employment problems; hypertensive or have vascular disease.

Investigating patients with possible OSAHS

Patients with possible OSAHS are mainly investigated during sleep, but some daytime tests have been used.

TESTS DURING WAKEFULNESS

An accurate test which would predict OSAHS in awake patients would be attractive. Various options have been explored, including the following.

Flow volume curves
Despite original suggestions that inspiratory flow volume curves might be a useful way to pick up upper airway narrowing and collapse during wakefulness in OSAHS, these have not proved to be useful diagnostically.[73,206]

Upper airway imaging
Neither acoustic reflection, CT nor MRI can accurately differentiate OSAHS patients from normal subjects by studying upper airway size or shape.[55,58–60,64]

Somnofluoroscopy
Direct visualization of the site of airway obstruction during sedation has been widely used by ENT surgeons to predict the occurrence and site of airway obstruction during sleep. However, there are no prospective correlational data showing that these measures reflect what happens during spontaneous sleep. Thus such studies cannot be recommended.

Facial structure

Retrognathia predisposes to OSAHS and jaw advancement is a possible treatment. It may be desirable to perform lateral cephalometry or facial CT imaging in non-obese patients found to have OSAHS.[62] This is particularly relevant in younger patients in whom surgical jaw advancement may be contemplated.

Thyroid function

Although there is an association between hypothyroidism and OSAHS, it is not cost-effective to screen all OSAHS patients for hypothyroidism.[207–209] The more rational approach is to check thyroid function in all suspected clinically of being hypothyroid.

TESTS DURING SLEEP

The principle requirement is a study of breathing during sleep. Patients should not be treated unless the diagnosis has been established. There is an ever-widening choice of equipment available to use for sleep studies and this book does not aim to advocate a 'best buy'. However, there are some general points which may be made.

Home sleep studies

Studies of breathing overnight at home allow patients to sleep in their own beds and thus perhaps sleep better than in a strange room in a sleep laboratory. Also, provided the equipment can be attached by the patient, home sleep studies are much cheaper than studies requiring the costs of a hospital bed.[210] If a technician needs to go to the patient's home to attach the equipment, this may be as expensive as a sleep laboratory study once travel time and costs are factored in. Thus, it is sensible to use simple monitoring for home studies and, although this is cost-efficient, it imposes limitations on the interpretation of the results. These include:

- Inability to tell whether the patient is awake or asleep. Fortunately, it is rare for patients with OSAHS who are usually somnolent to fail to sleep at home, but this possibility must be remembered if a home study is unexpectedly normal. The lack of documentation of sleep equally causes a problem because respiratory events during wakefulness are included in the overall score,[211] whereas these would be excluded in a study recording sleep.
- Many home systems use suboptimal sensors to detect respiratory events. This is particularly true for 'flow' sensors which are often temperature sensors and thus poor at identifying hypopnoeas.[15] Sensors for thoraco-

abdominal movement are often different from those used in polysomnography with different sensitivities and this must be appreciated when the results are interpreted. More basic oximeters are also used on some systems and may be less reliable.

- Inability to detect diagnoses other than OSAHS. Most systems cannot identify arousals and thus no clues will be given to the periodic limb movement disorder. Similarly, although overnight sleep studies never provide a firm diagnosis of narcolepsy, home systems will not provide evidence of early REM sleep and sleep disturbance which may provide clues.

It is critical that all such studies are interpreted by individuals trained in sleep medicine and aware of the limitations of the device used. One of the biggest problems with OSAHS diagnosis is that untrained individuals blindly believe the numbers derived by (often unvalidated) software without realizing the potential pitfalls.

Provided these limitations are appreciated, home sleep studies are very useful, cost-effective and convenient for patients and can significantly speed up investigation of patients with possible OSAHS.[210] I believe in-hospital sleep studies will soon be the first overnight investigation for only a small minority of patients. However, sleepy patients with a normal home limited sleep study **must** proceed to further investigation as a normal overnight limited sleep study could be due to inadequate sleep, inadequate sensors or to there being a non-OSAHS cause for the patient's sleepiness.

It has been suggested that patients diagnosed with limited sleep studies have poorer CPAP use thereafter.[212] This is not our experience[210] nor can we understand any reason why this might be so if the CPAP education process is carefully carried out.

In-hospital limited sleep studies

The same limited sleep study equipment can be used in the hospital setting where it has the same ability to make a diagnosis of OSAHS if positive, but polysomnography is required if a limited study is negative in a sleepy patient. The cost benefit of performing limited studies in hospital is dubious as the space used may be as expensive as that for polysomnography and the savings in staff and equipment costs need to be set against the costs of repeating inconclusive studies.

Polysomnography

Studies which record sleep and breathing became known in the USA as polysomnography, or psg, even although many 'limited sleep study' systems which do not record sleep also result in multiple (poly) channels during sleep (somno) being recorded (graph). Polysomnography was originally always performed in a sleep laboratory but, as a result of improved electronics and data storage, can now be performed in the home as well. However, the costs of home polysomnography exceed those for in laboratory studies because a technician generally needs to travel to the home to set up the patient, so home psg is usually only done for research rather than clinical studies.

There are major differences in polysomnographic techniques between sleep centres which must be appreciated when evaluating results. Many result from the use of different sensors and some from the use of different definitions of events. It is vital these differences are appreciated.

SENSORS

'Flow'

Sensors to detect apnoeas were usually thermocouples or thermisters designed to detect 'flow' by the difference between the warm exhaled air and the cooler inhaled air. Although these are excellent apnoea detectors, the signal is not quantitative as 50 ml of expired air has virtually the same temperature as 500 ml of expired air. More accurate quantification can be obtained by recording either true respired volume by use of a sealed facemask and pneumotachograph – rarely used because it is cumbersome – or nasal pressure.[213] Nasal pressure provides quantitative measure of nasal flow but will not necessary provide a good measure of overall flow when there is mouth breathing. Thankfully, pure mouth breathing is unusual during sleep[214] and when partial mouth breathing occurs the nasal pressure signal is usually still adequate to allow scoring. Further data are required to clarify how often scoring of flow from nasal pressure is made uncertain by mouth breathing although initial estimates of nine per cent of studies seem high[215] compared to other data.[214]

At present I would advocate the use of nasal pressure as the best flow sensor, with simultaneous use of a thermocouple in front of the mouth to detect whether mouth breathing is occurring, but this is a rapidly moving field. Nasal pressure is the measurement recommended by the American Academy of Sleep Medicine Task Force,[16] although thermal sensors are adequate apnoea sensors provided they are not used to estimate hypopnoeas.[15]

'Thoraco-abdominal movement'

Conventionally, some measure of thoracic and/or abdominal movement has been recorded, and this was originally designed to differentiate central from obstructive apnoeas. However, it is now recognized that:

● Many apnoeas in which no thoraco-abdominal movement may be detected are actually obstructive. Identification of chest wall movement is particularly difficult in the very obese.

- Central apnoeas can only be identified with if either oesophageal pressure[16] or respiratory muscle electromyography is recorded and absent during the events.

The current rationale for recording thoraco-abdominal movement is to provide a semi-quantitative measure of respired volume to detect hypopnoeas.[15] The current recommendation of the American Academy of Sleep Medicine Task Force[16] is that both nasal pressure and thoraco-abdominal movement by inductance plethysmography should be recorded to allow redundancy and certainty in the detection of hypopnoeas.

'Airflow obstruction'

Episodes of partial obstruction of the airway may be detected by recording oesophageal pressure directly[17,216] or indirectly,[217] flow limitation[218,219] or by measuring airways resistance.[220] Each has advantages and disadvantages.

Recording oesophageal pressure is relatively invasive and can only be performed in a sleep laboratory, adding to the costs. Swallowing oesophageal catheters does not appeal to all patients and the presence of such a catheter may disturb sleep, although less in a sleepy patient than in a normal subject. Pressure may be recorded by use of an oesophageal balloon, a water-filled catheter or a catheter-mounted pressure transducer system.[17,216] Analysis of the oesophageal pressure signal on its own is insufficient to detect episodes of airflow obstruction as oesophageal pressure swings may rise due to either increased resistance or increased flow. Thus, both flow and oesophageal pressure must be inspected together and ideally the ratio pressure/flow computed on a breath-by-breath basis. All this makes recording of oesophageal pressure on a routine basis unattractive.

Pleural pressure swings can also be assessed non-invasively from the resulting changes in arterial blood pressure.[217] Unfortunately, current technology does not allow the non-invasive measurement of beat-to-beat blood pressure without disturbing sleep. Both the Finapress device[97] and, to a lesser extent, the Portapress which use finger plethysmography to record blood pressure become uncomfortable after some hours of use and thus disturb sleep. A measure of blood pressure may be obtained from measurement of the speed of propagation of the pulse wave from the heart to the periphery – the pulse transit time or PTT.[221] The pulse wave travels faster the higher the pressure and so the shorter the PTT the higher the blood pressure. Thus, episodes of increased airflow obstruction associated with a more negative intra-thoracic pressure will be associated with a more negative intra-cardiac pressure and thus a slower PTT.[222] Preliminary results suggest this may be a useful non-invasive measure of episodes of airflow obstruction.[221,223] PTT can be derived from the interval between the R wave on the electrocardiograph and the arrival of the pulse wave at the finger as detected by an oximeter probe. As with direct measurement of oesophageal pressure, PTT should be viewed in conjunction with the flow signal to judge whether changes are due to changes in flow or resistance.

On inspiration, the upper airway acts as a floppy tube with the characteristics of a Starling resistor during sleep. Thus, the inspiratory flow rate becomes independent of the respiratory effort and is limited by partial collapse of the pharynx at a stage before the airway actually occludes. In practice this is best seen as flattening of the mid-portion of the flow/time plot (Figure 2.15). Such flow limitation may be identified either visually[218,219] or automatically[224] and can be used as a marker of episodes of increased airflow resistance. The specificity and sensitivity of episodes of flow limitation needs further study, but there is no doubt that the recognition of the characteristic flattening shape is at worst a useful adjunct in recognizing resistive episodes and at best may make the measurement of oesophageal pressure redundant.[219]

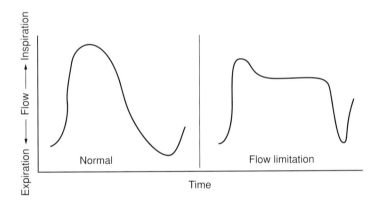

Figure 2.15
Flow time curves with normal breathing and with flow limitation during upper airway narrowing on inspiration.

Airflow resistance has been measured directly during sleep studies by the forced oscillation technique.[220] This technique requires the patient to wear a facemask with no leak and its applicability in diagnosis is uncertain. However, this is a useful method of determining whether events occurring on CPAP are associated with airway narrowing.[224,225]

Snoring

It is useful to be able to record snoring to determine whether:

● Patients with apnoeas and hypopnoeas snore around the time of the events adding strong support to an obstructive aetiology.

- Patients who report snoring but do not turn out to have OSAHS snore sufficiently to warrant therapy aimed at their snoring. Many patients who present with intolerable habitual snoring are found to snore rarely if at all.

Snoring can be recorded by use of a microphone or derived from the nasal pressure signal.

Sleep

The presence and type of sleep is classically determined by recording a combination of the electro-encephalogram (EEG), electro-oculogram (EOG) and electro-myogram (EMG). Sleep is usually staged by visual inspection applying rules derived by Rechtschaffen and Kales in 1968[226] which score each 30-second period into one of six categories according to the frequency of the underlying neurophysiological signals. The key components of the scoring system are discussed in Chapter 1. The same signals may be examined to detect brief awakenings from sleep, usually called arousals or micro-arousals[227] which are discussed in Chapter 1.

Value of sleep scoring in the investigation of patients with possible OSAHS

Scoring sleep stages is certainly not essential to diagnose most patients with OSAHS. Patients with recurrent apnoeas or hypopnoeas overnight can be diagnosed readily without knowledge of sleep stage, especially if they are associated with recurrent desaturation. The neurophysiological signals give no additional clues to the diagnosis.[228] It may be helpful to know whether a patient is awake or asleep for two reasons:

- Rarely, patients with OSAHS may fail to sleep well or at all on a diagnostic night and thus the diagnosis may be missed or the severity underestimated if there is no knowledge of sleep duration.
- Patients who have a normal breathing pattern during sleep may occasionally be diagnosed as having sleep apnoea if breath-holding events during wakefulness – often associated with restlessness – are falsely attributed to sleep.

However, sleep duration may be recorded in other, non-neurophysiological, ways. Lack of movement is a basic characteristic of sleep and can be used to estimate sleep duration from an activity monitor attached to the arm,[229,230] a static charged bed[214] or from video recording. Although none is as accurate at assessing sleep duration as neurophysiological scoring, all are much cheaper both in terms of capital and staff costs, and are less inconvenient for the patient. Further data on their efficacy in monitoring sleep duration in patients with OSAHS is required.

Scoring of arousals from the neurophysiological signals can be very time-consuming. It is doubtful whether routine scoring of arousals from electro-physiological signals during all sleep studies is worthwhile as:

- In cases where there is clear abnormality of breathing, scoring arousals does not allow more accurate prediction of treatment benefit compared to simpler ways of detecting arousals.[103]
- Recurrent brief 'arousals' induced by sound can be characterized by changes in blood pressure and result in sleepiness without there being sufficient neurophysiological change to score arousals.[102] Thus the ASDA definition of arousals[227] is missing clinically important events.
- The reproducibility of scoring arousals from EEG may be highly variable between sleep centres,[231] although more reliable within centres.[232]

Possible ways of detecting arousals non-electrophysiologically include recording the arousal associated increases in:

- Heart rate.
- Blood pressure measured by finger plethysmography.[102]
- Blood pressure inferred from a decrease in pulse transit time.[221,223]
- Tidal volume that occurs with arousal.[211]

It is not yet clear which approach is best or whether scoring of non-electrophysiological arousals is diagnostically or therapeutically useful, but it is likely that they will have a role at least in diagnosis. At present, evidence of an increased arousal frequency is useful in two situations; first, when breathing is normal and thus sleep disruption due to a non-respiratory cause needs to be considered in sleepy patients, and second, when breathing pattern changes do not reach diagnostic thresholds in sleepy patients and the diagnosis of the upper airways resistance syndrome has to be considered.[17,19]

Oxygen saturation

Oxygenation is measured by oximetry which senses the colour and hence oxygen saturation of the arterial blood arriving with each pulse. Usually this is recorded by use of a probe on the finger, although other vascular structures including the ear may be used and in some cases may be more accurate. Oximeters have limitations to their accuracy and time response which vary between instruments and users must be aware of the characteristics of their oximeter. Many will measure oxygen saturation to an accuracy of approximately ±3 per cent between individuals,[233] although the accuracy within individuals may be greater. All become less reliable if perfusion is poor, and this can sometimes be a problem if patients lie on the instrumented part. Overnight oxygen saturation traces can be diagnostic in some patients[228] (Figure 2.16).

Figure 2.16
Overnight oxygen saturation during sleep in a patient with OSAHS and an apnoea/hypopnoea index (AHI) of 60 per hour.

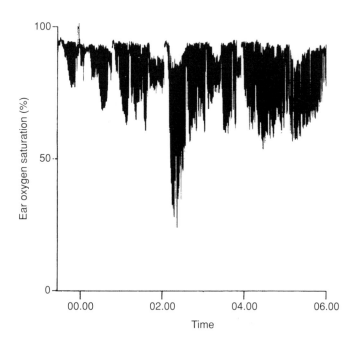

Heart rate

Heart rate may be used to help detect arousals and can be recorded from pulse oximetry or from ECG. In many centres ECG is recorded routinely during polysomnography. Although cardiac arrhythmias are commonly found during the night, their clinical significance is unknown and it is likely that any such arrhythmia has been occurring frequently on non-monitored nights.

Position

Body position influences snoring and AHI in many patients and it is useful to know whether patients sleep on their back and whether events only happened when they were supine. Position is usually measured by piezo-electric or mercury tilt systems.

What type of sleep study – polysomnography or limited recording?

Recording of multiple channels, including EEG, in a sleep laboratory (Figure 2.17) was the standard way to diagnose sleep apnoea and remains so in many parts of the world. However, this approach has been questioned[228,234] because:

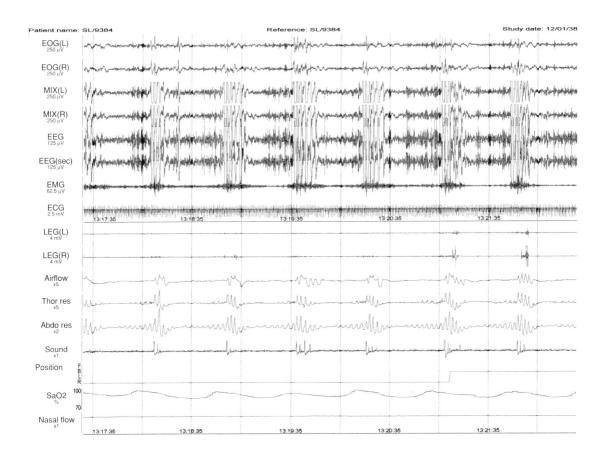

Figure 2.17
Polysomnography recording
showing a five-minute
period with seven
obstructive apnoeas each
associated with snoring and
an arousal.

- It is expensive in terms of hospital space, equipment and staff.
- Simpler approaches are sufficient in many patients.
- Studies done in the patient's home are usually cheaper.
- Sleep will not be normal in a strange bedroom with a large amount of monitoring equipment, and patients may also lie on their back more. Both sleep disturbance and the supine posture may result in overestimation of irregular breathing during sleep.

On the other hand, polysomnography has some advantages in terms of:

- Certainty whether the patient slept.
- Identification of artefact.
- Use of better sensors with built-in redundancy.

The investigational approach used will vary between sleep centres, depending on the facilities available, their costs and patients' travel distances. Our practice is to perform home studies on all local patients with patients applying the equipment to themselves at home and collecting and returning it. However, distant patients come in for polysomnography as do local patients with strongly suggestive symptoms but equivocal home studies. This approach has been validated and found to be cost-effective.[210]

The advantages and disadvantages of different diagnostic approaches are discussed more fully in Chapter 5.

Treatment

WHO TO TREAT FOR OSAHS?

Current evidence from randomized controlled trials indicates that objective improvements with treatment may be found in symptomatic patients with more than 10 respiratory events per hour.[135,235] These benefits are in daytime alertness and sleepiness. Treatment should thus be focused on these benefits and not given in the hope of diminishing vascular risk in asymptomatic patients, for whom there is no evidence of benefit from randomised controlled trials at present.[236]

GENERAL MEASURES

All patients with OSAHS should have the mechanism and significance of the condition explained to them and preferably to their partners as well. This should be done using a combined approach involving doctors, nurses and written and video material. Patients and their partners have to commit to life-long treatment and must understand why.

Overweight patients should be asked to lose weight as weight reduction improves OSAHS.[237] Unfortunately, sustained weight loss is not often achieved whatever resources are applied, but it should always be sought. The role of gastro-intestinal surgery in weight reduction in the morbidly obese OSAHS patient remains under debate, but this should certainly be considered in appropriate patients.[238] However, even after surgically induced sustained weight loss, recurrence of OSAHS has been reported.[239]

Patients who smoke should be asked to stop. Although there is epidemiological data linking smoking with OSAHS[23] there is no evidence stopping smoking improves OSAHS. Indeed, stopping smoking is often associated with weight gain which may worsen OSAHS. I thus do not focus on smoking except in non-obese patients.

Patients should be advised to avoid alcohol in the evenings and not to use sleeping tablets or sedatives. All decrease upper airway dilating muscle function and worsen OSAHS.

These general steps may suffice in simple snorers or those with few symptoms and mild OSAHS, but most will require additional treatment.

CPAP

CPAP therapy for sleep apnoea was originally proposed by Sullivan in 1981[13] as a temporary treatment for OSAHS until something better was found. We are still waiting! CPAP acts by raising the pressure within the upper airway to a high enough level to force the throat open during sleep and prevent it being sucked closed (Figure 2.18).

CPAP is the treatment of OSAHS with the firmest evidence base[240,241] despite earlier scepticism.[242] Randomized controlled trials show that CPAP improves symptoms, subjective and objective sleepiness,[134,135,191,243] cognitive function, vigilance, mood[135,191] and quality of life[135,235,244] in OSAHS patients. Unequivocal objective improvements are found in symptomatic patients with more than 15 apnoeas plus hypopnoeas per hour slept[135] or more than 10 four per cent desaturations per hour.[235]

Prospective studies have also found that CPAP improves OSAHS patients' performance on driving simulators[125,126] and decreases the frequency and severity of road accidents.[127,128,245,246]

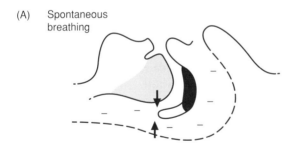

(A)   Spontaneous breathing

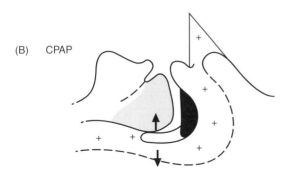

(B)   CPAP

Figure 2.18
Schematic of (A) suction causing apnoeas and (B) CPAP blowing the upper airway open.

Randomized controlled studies[159,247] have also shown that CPAP reduces 24-hour blood pressure in symptomatic patient with an AHI greater than 15 per hour. Most of this effect is on night-time blood pressure. On average, 24-hour diastolic pressure fell by 1.5 mm Hg with CPAP when analysed on an intention to treat basis with a 5 mm Hg fall in diastolic and 4 mm Hg fall in systolic pressure in patients with significant hypoxaemia during sleep, defined a priori as more than 20 four per cent desaturations per hour.[159] The BP drop was also greater in those that used CPAP most.

In milder patients (AHI 5–15 per hour), the benefits of CPAP are statistically significant in randomized controlled trials but only in terms of subjective outcomes[134,248] and thus further studies are required before CPAP can be recommended as standard treatment for this group. This is particularly the case as long-term use of CPAP in mild patients is poor[249] with only 50 per cent of those with an AHI of less than 15 per hour still using CPAP at three years.

Starting CPAP therapy

Initiating treatment with CPAP is a vitally important process to ensure success and must involve:

- Education of patients, preferably along with their partner, about the rationale for CPAP and the need for long-term treatment. This should be undertaken before the night of the CPAP trial to allow adequate time for discussion and to allow patients to adjust to the concept.
- Fitting patients with the most comfortable mask system for them. This should involve trials with multiple masks for several different manufacturers because different masks fit different patients best.
- Giving patients an opportunity to try CPAP when awake so they understand what is involved before using it at night.
- A night-time study to set the appropriate CPAP pressure; one high enough to minimize respiratory events, but low enough to permit sleep.
- Careful follow-up and support for patients, particularly in the early days of treatment. We provide a 24-hour phone help line and encourage early reporting of problems.

The more intensive this education and support process, the better are the CPAP use and outcomes achieved.[250,251] Hoy and colleagues[251] showed that better CPAP usage and outcomes were achieved if the CPAP education involved partners as well as patients, patients were kept in the sleep centre for three nights at CPAP initiation to troubleshoot problems and were followed up frequently with home visits by specialist CPAP nurses. Which of these elements made the difference is unknown but my belief is that involving partners might have been the key element.

CPAP titration

Initially, CPAP pressures were set by manual adjustment of the pressure while watching the patient's breathing and sleep patterns. Usually the goal of the titration was to abolish apnoeas and minimize hypopnoeas and arousals whilst ensuring good quality sleep. Too high a pressure will prevent sleep and too low a pressure will not abolish significant respiratory events. Such manual titration is successful but expensive in terms of staff time and equipment and requires full polysomnography. There was not a good correlation between the physiological success of a CPAP trial and the outcome of CPAP therapy.[252]

Intelligent CPAP machines which automatically adjust the CPAP pressure in response to apnoeas, hyopopnoeas, increased air flow resistance or snoring are now widely used to determine what level of CPAP patients need.[253–255] We have used intelligent CPAP machines in our sleep centre for the vast majority of CPAP titration studies for the past five years, and no longer record sleep during titration studies.

Split-night studies

Traditionally, CPAP titration studies always involved a whole night study in a sleep centre. However, the need to decrease costs has lead to many centres performing a diagnostic test in the first part of the night and if that shows clear OSAHS then a CPAP titration is performed during the rest of the night.[256–259]

Our practice is to reserve split-night studies for those whose histories strongly suggest OSAHS, and to educate them for CPAP and fit them for masks prior to the night-time study. Split-night studies are performed allowing at least two hours for the diagnostic component. If, after two hours, the technician or nurse is confident that the AHI is more than 20 per hour, the rest of the night will be a CPAP titration study.[259] If the staff are not confident at two hours that the AHI is more than 20 per hour the whole night is used as a diagnostic study. Using this protocol we have found similar long-term CPAP use and patient outcomes as with whole-night CPAP trials following a whole-night diagnostic study.[259]

Home CPAP therapy

After the initiation of CPAP, patients should be given as much support as possible by trained CPAP nurses or technicians. Because CPAP use in the first few days is the strongest predictor of long-term use[260] our CPAP nurses telephone patients after their first night at home on CPAP to try to troubleshoot any problems rapidly. Patients are then followed up as required by telephone and have access to a 24-hour helpline.

CPAP use

Patients use all long-term medication less than their doctors wish, with acceptable use in only approximately 60 per cent in asthma[261] and hypertension.[262] CPAP is no exception. Many patients use CPAP much less than requested by their doctors, and some not at all. Thus CPAP use must be monitored in all patients.

Patients overestimate their use in comparison to objectively measured machine run times,[263,264] and thus patient use times are not reliable.[265] Objective CPAP can be recorded most simply by measuring the time that the CPAP machine is switched on. This gives a time which is much closer to actual use than are patients' reports.[263,264] However, these 'run times' will include time when the mask has been taken off in the middle of the night and also times when the machine is switched on in another room if the patient aims to mislead. Thus, in patients in whom use must be assessed accurately, a device measuring the time that the patient is breathing on the CPAP machine should be used.[263,264] Most manufacturers have such devices and software. It would be reasonable to make these systems mandatory for all professional drivers on CPAP and for others working in potentially dangerous environments. They should also be used in all research studies.

Average CPAP use in a group of patients will vary depending on selection criteria. In a group of unselected OSAHS patients started on CPAP, and including non-users in the analysis, average 'run time' is approximately three to four hours a night.[134,191,248,266] In a group of patients attending a CPAP users clinic then average 'run time' will be five hours or more per night[267,268] as the non-users and low users will have dropped out.

In some centres, up to 50 per cent of patients refuse to start on CPAP,[269] whereas this figure is less than five per cent in our centre.[249] This may reflect differences in patient selection, education, support and costs to patients.

Predictors of CPAP use

The best correlates of long term CPAP use[249] are AHI, Epworth sleepiness score and presence of snoring. Ninety-four per cent of patients with an AHI of more than 30 and an ESS of more than 15 will still be using CPAP at five years[249] (Figure 2.19). In contrast only 25 per cent of those with an AHI of less than 15 per hour and an ESS less than 11 will be using CPAP by five years.

Other factors which can predict use include whether the patient self-initiated the referral[251] and higher BMI,[249,268] but this may reflect the interaction between BMI and AHI as BMI was not a significant factor in a multivariate analysis.[249] Younger patients and those without co-existing lung disease tend to use CPAP better.[249,268]

The strongest predictor of long term use is initial CPAP use. Use at four days predicts use at two months[260] and that at four weeks predicts use at three

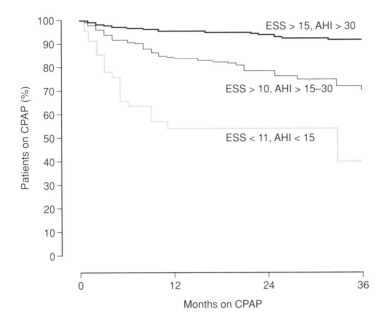

Figure 2.19
Effect of sleepiness (Epworth sleepiness score, ESS) and incidence of apnoea/hypopnoea (AHI) on the percentage of patients continuing to use CPAP. (Adapted from McArdle *et al.*,[249] with permission.)

months.[270] In addition, use in the first three months is the best predictor of long-term CPAP use.[249]

Side-effects of CPAP

CPAP has downsides.[267] Major life-threatening side-effects are rare, although pneumocephalus has been reported.[271] The more usual problems are:

- The concept of sleeping with a mask is unacceptable to some, particularly those with claustrophobia. Intranasal 'pillows' systems may be better for some of these.
- Discomfort from the mask, which can usually be resolved by trying enough masks from a range of makers. Mask design is improving considerably but ideal comfort is still not always achievable.
- Nasal symptoms, including stuffiness, rhinitis and drying, occur in approximately 60 per cent of CPAP users and are major problems in at least four per cent.[267] Nasal symptoms are usually due to mouth leaks causing high flows of cool air through the nose[272] and attempts should be made to reduce these either by chin straps or full facemasks. However, CPAP use with the early full facemasks was less than with nasal masks[273] and many patients find them inconvenient. In a few patients intranasal steroids may help. However, for many a heated humidifier to add to their CPAP system appears to be the best solution.[272,274]
- Abdominal bloating can occur but in our experience is rarely troublesome, being a major problem in less than one per cent.[267]

It is unclear whether intelligent CPAP systems which vary the pressure overnight to normalize breathing will have fewer side-effects and better outcomes than conventional fixed pressure systems. Preliminary data suggest they may.[275]

CPAP follow-up

Protocols will vary between centres. The essential requirement is that the patients have ready access to trained CPAP support workers. In our centre, as well as the early telephone call from the CPAP nurses and access to a 24-hour helpline, patients are followed up in a nurse-led clinic at two, six and 12 months. Visits are moved to annually thereafter unless problems intervene. All the CPAP units provided have built-in 'run time' clocks and these are read at each visit and daily use is computed. If CPAP use is less than four hours a night, problems limiting CPAP use are sought and rectified if possible. If use is less than two hours a night patients are warned that continued poor use will result in repossession of the CPAP machine by the sleep centre. Repossession occurs in approximately 5–10 per cent of cases.

Home use of intelligent CPAP systems

Intelligent CPAP machines which increase the pressure as required can be used successfully long term.[276,277] Theoretically, these machines could be more comfortable, as the pressure will be lower when the patient is awake, and could have fewer side-effects, as the flow through the mask – and thus nasal symptoms – might be lower. There is some evidence that this may be the case[275,277] and that outcomes may be improved.[275]

Intelligent CPAP machines made by different manufacturers differ markedly in their mode of action. This field is evolving so rapidly that readers are encouraged to consult recent literature.

Bi-level ventilation for OSAHS

In some centres, bi-level ventilators are used instead of CPAP for some patients. These devices allow independent adjustment of inspiratory and expiratory pressures rather than having the same pressure for both as CPAP does. Bi-level ventilators are effective but they are much more expensive than CPAP machines – about six times the price – and there is no good evidence that they produce better outcomes than CPAP. A well-designed prospective study found no advantage for bi-level ventilators over conventional CPAP.[278]

DENTAL SPLINTING

OSAHS is caused by the throat narrowing during sleep, at least partly due to the tongue being sucked back and the jaw dropping open and backwards when muscle tone drops during sleep. Mandibular repositioning splints (MRSs) are designed to keep the lower jaw, and thus the tongue, forward so preventing the throat narrowing.

There is randomized controlled trial evidence that mandibular advancement splints can decrease snoring[279] in simple snorers and improve symptoms and overnight breathing patterns in patients with mild OSAHS.[280–282] Thus far, there are few data comparing the efficacy of one type of MRS device against another. Devices differ in many ways, including the degree of jaw advancement and whether this is adjustable, the extent of mouth opening produced, the rigidity of the tooth fixation system and whether lateral jaw movement is possible.[282] The relative merits and disadvantages of the different designs are poorly documented, although comparative studies are emerging.[283] This study suggests that simpler single block constructed devices may sometimes be better in terms of patient preference for symptom relief and simplicity of use, although objective breathing during sleep was similar on the mono-bloc and Herbst devices.[283]

Side-effects of MRS devices vary between series, but in general, minor side-effects are very common but severe ones rare. In one series of 130 patients, three-quarters of subjects had side-effects, including excess salivation, xerostomia, temporo-mandibular joint pain, dental discomfort and myofacial discomfort, each of which occurred in around a quarter of patients,[284] but only seven per cent reported ceasing treatment because of severe side-effects.

As yet there are no adequate randomized controlled trials of MRSs against CPAP in patients with OSAHS. The existing studies suggest that patients tend to prefer MRSs[280,281] but objective data suggest that outcomes may be better for CPAP in terms of breathing during sleep and daytime function.[285] Patients' preference for MRSs is important, but it is not known whether this means they feel better on MRSs or that they find the concept of an non-obtrusive intra-oral device preferable to use of an obtrusive CPAP device.

Mandibular repositioning splints at present are the second line therapy of choice for patients with mild to moderate sleep apnoea who will not tolerate CPAP. However, this is an evolving area and advances in device design may alter this position. Among the areas to be resolved are: what are the best MRS devices?; does the best device vary between patients?; how to assess the degree of advancement required; what are the long-term benefits and side-effects?; and what is the long-term objective use of MRS devices?

It is unclear whether CPAP or MRSs have the greater cost–benefit utility. The basic cost of many MRS devices is less than the cost of a CPAP machine, but this is by no means true for all devices – adjustable MRSs tend to be expensive. Further, orthodontic charges may be high with multiple visits needed to adjust some of the devices. Also, in some studies at least, the time taken to adjust the MRS device to optimal performance was much longer (more than six months) than the one night usually needed for CPAP titration.

Thus, the role of MRS devices is evolving. I believe they are the best second-line therapy available for OSAHS if CPAP is not tolerated.

SURGERY

A single operation has major attractions over nightly therapy for life, particularly for younger patients. Many surgical treatments for OSAHS have been tried but few evaluated rigorously.

Uvulopalatopharyngoplasty

Probably the most widely performed operation has been the uvulopalatopharyngoplasty, usually known as UPPP or U3P. There are many variants, but all attempt to widen the retropalatal airway by removing the uvula and part of the soft palate combined with tensing the lateral pharyngeal walls.[286] Early studies reported significant improvements in symptoms and some improvement in breathing during sleep. However:

- None had adequate control groups and none were randomized.[90]
- Complications of UPPP are poorly documented in most studies. Deaths have occurred.[90,286,287]
- The degree of improvement in breathing abnormality was usually much less than with CPAP.[90,286]
- Many studies classified as successes patients who still had a pathological breathing pattern during sleep.[286]
- Follow-up studies report that improvement is not sustained[288] with many patients needing additional therapy in terms of CPAP or maxillofacial surgery, particularly if they gain weight.[289]
- Patients who fail to benefit from UPPP often have difficulty coping with CPAP as there is no longer a good seal between the palate and the tongue. Thus the pressure applied to the nose tends to leak out of the mouth, decreasing efficacy and causing discomfort and side-effects.[290]
- Two recent reviews have concluded that there is no current evidence to support the use of this operation to try to cure OSAHS.[90,286]

These comments apply equally to the procedure whether it is carried out using a scalpel, laser (LAUP) or diathermy. The American Sleep Disorders Association (ASDA) concluded in 1994 that 'LAUP is not recommended for the treatment of sleep related breathing disorders'. Since then studies have shown LAUP to change mean AHI from 29 to 22 per hour[291] and, in another, LAUP had no effect on AHI once allowance had been made for weight loss.[292]

Attempts have been made to improve the response rate to UPPP by identifying the site of obstruction by CT, MRI or endoscopic visualization under sedation and only operating on palatal obstructors. This has resulted in some evidence of higher success rates.[286] However, the studies analysed were not controlled and the retropalatal obstructors had less severe AHIs pre-operatively, whereas the response rate overall was inversely proportional to AHI. Further, the overall decrease in AHI was similar in these retropalatal obstructors (33 per cent, standard deviation (SD) 61 per cent) to those in whom no attempt was made to localize the site of obstruction (32 per cent, SD 58 per cent). Thus the benefits of localizing the site of obstruction before UPPP are unclear and probably limited.

Side-effects of UPPP include:

- Death in at least 16 cases.[286]
- Considerable pain in the immediate post-operative period.
- Velopharyngeal insufficiency found in 39 per cent of patients at two years when rigorous steps were taken to identify it.[293] This is often asymptomatic but 24 per cent of patients report symptomatic reflux at one year.[294]
- Voice change may occur but the frequency is unclear.

Despite all these concerns there is no doubt the operation can help some patients with objective improvements in AHI and in other outcomes such as driving ability.[295] Carefully conducted randomized controlled trials are needed to establish whether there is both subjective and objective benefit of UPPP in pre-selected patient groups and whether these improvements are sustained.[90,286,287] A 'one off' operation has considerable advantages over nightly therapy, particularly for younger patients, but UPPP cannot be recommended on the basis of current evidence.

OTHER UPPER AIRWAY SURGERY

In a few specialist centres, mainly in North America, surgery has been also aimed at widening the airway behind the tongue by:

- Debulking the base of the tongue. Laser mid-line glossectomy has been reported to help 40 per dent of OSAHS patients.[296] The same group has reported a 77 per cent success rate with the relatively extensive operation of lingualplasty.[297]
- Advancing the insertion of the tongue by advancing the genial tubercle of the mandible.[298] This may be combined with altering the position of the hyoid bone.

These procedures which are often staged may be effective in the majority of patients in highly specialized surgical hands.[299]

Nasal surgery

Patients with OSAHS are frequently referred for nasal surgery in the logical belief that nasal obstruction will predispose to more negative intra-pharyngeal pressure during inspiration and thus obstructive apnoeas. However, evidence that procedures such as polypectomy or submucous resection help OSAHS does not exist.[300]

Radiofrequency volume reduction

There has been a recent vogue for treating OSAHS and snoring with radiofrequency volume reduction of the tongue or soft palate. Although this works in animal models[301] and may reduce snoring and sleep apnoea in the short term in uncontrolled studies,[302,303] there are doubts about the long-term efficacy.[304] This treatment cannot be advised at present.

Mandibulo-maxillary osteotomy

Advancement of the mandible and maxilla by cutting both at an angle and rejoining them after sliding them forward (Figure 2.20) is more major surgery.[305,306] However, this procedure is regularly performed by maxillofacial surgery for other conditions. Mandibulo-maxillary osteotomy (MMO) has been shown in a controlled trial to be as effective as CPAP in

Figure 2.20
Maxillo-mandibular osteotomy with rigid plate fixation of maxilla and screw fixation of bilateral sagittal split mandibular osteomy.

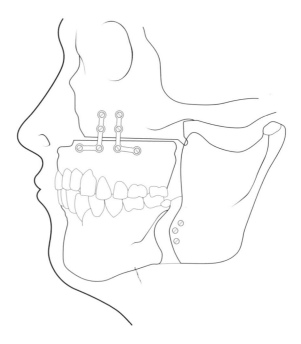

normalizing breathing pattern overnight and improving both symptoms and daytime vigilance.[307] The precise indications for MMO are not yet clear and specifically whether minor retro-position of the mandible and maxilla are prerequisites for this approach. However, provided experienced surgeons are available, MMO should be considered in:

- Younger patients who are not grossly obese.
- Patients with severe OSAHS who decline CPAP therapy.

Long-term results seem good with 12/15 severe patients having an AHI of less than 10 per hour at two years[308] and a mean AHI of nine (SD 6) per hour at six months.[309]

Pacing

Attempts have been made to treat OSAHS by pacing the tongue when upper airway obstruction occurs during sleep.[310] There is no doubt that this approach can reduce apnoeas, but the long-term results are unknown and the technical challenges are formidable. Not least among these is the large number of muscles that participate in the development of upper airway obstruction.

Medication

Unfortunately, there is no good evidence of benefit of any drug therapy as sole treatment for human OSAHS. Drugs tried include REM suppressants – protriptyline – acetazolamide and progesterone, but there are no adequate controlled trials showing clinical benefit.[311] Indeed, side-effects outweigh benefits for all these agents. There is some evidence that the addition of stimulant drugs to CPAP may have a small beneficial effect in patients remaining sleepy despite using their CPAP, but concern that CPAP use may be reduced causing a potential increase in vascular risk.[312]

At present, trials are underway with adenosine and serotonin-related drugs. There is some evidence of partial efficacy of ondansetron, a serotonin$_3$ antagonist[313] on improving breathing during sleep in bulldogs.

COST/BENEFIT ANALYSIS

Patients with undiagnosed OSAHS are heavy users of healthcare.[314] Indeed, healthcare expenditure on undiagnosed OSAHS patients is around twice that of age- and gender-matched control subjects[314,315] and this difference extends back over 10 years prior to the diagnosis of OSAHS being made.[316] The increased costs average approximately US $1300/patient year.[315]

Treatment of OSAHS with CPAP reduces these costs with evidence of decreased hospitalization with cardiovascular and pulmonary disease[317] and decreased hospital stays due to road accidents.[127] Overall, mean hospitalization days/year decreased with CPAP therapy.[318] The size of the saving to healthcare budgets of treating patients with OSAHS needs to be clarified by further large scale studies, although the fact that there is a saving is clear.[245,318]

There is also a need for more studies on the cost utility of CPAP and other treatments. One study has estimated that CPAP resulted in an average gain of 5.4 quality adjusted life years (QALYs) at a cost of 3400–9800 Canadian dollars/QALY added,[319] equivalent to £1500–4400 or US$2200–6300. Another estimate largely based on Jenkinson's study[235] suggests approximately £3200 (US $4600)/QALY added.[320] These are cost levels which would strongly justify treatment, but more studies are needed.

References

1 Kryger, M.H. (1983) Sleep apnea. From the needles of Dionysius to continuous positive airway pressure. *Arch. Intern. Med.*, **143**, 2301–3.

2 Lavie, P. (1984) Nothing new under the moon. Historical accounts of sleep apnea syndrome. *Arch. Intern. Med.*, **144**, 2025–8.

3 Wadd, W. (1829) Cursory remarks on corpulence. London: John Ebers & Co.

4 Dickens, C. (1836) *The Posthumous Papers of the Pickwick Club.* London: Chapman & Hall.

5 Broadbent, W.H. (1877) Cheyne–Stokes respiration in cerebral haemorrhage. *Lancet*, **1**, 307–9.

6 Caton, R. (1889) Case of narcolepsy. *Clin. Soc. Trans.*, **22**, 133–7.

7 Morison, A. (1889) Somnolence with cyanosis cured by massage. *Practitioner*, **42**, 277–81.

8 Spitz, A. (1937) Das klinische syndrome: Narcolepsy mit Fettsucht und Polyglobuliein seinem Beziehungen zum morbus Cushing. *Deutsch Arch. Klin. Med.*, **181**, 286.

9 Burwell, C.S., Robin, E.D., Whaley, R.D., Bickelmann, A.G. (1956) Extreme obesity associated with alveolar hypoventilation – a Pickwickian syndrome. *Am. J. Med.*, **21**, 811–18.

10 Jung, R., Kuhlo, W. (1965) Neurophysiological studies of abnormal night sleep and the Pickwickian syndrome in sleep mechanisms. *Prog. Brain Res.*, **18**, 140–60.

11 Gastaut, H., Tassinari, C.A., Duron, B. (1965) [Polygraphic study of diurnal and nocturnal (hypnic and respiratory) episodal manifestations of Pickwick syndrome]. *Rev. Neurol.* (Paris), **112**, 568–79.

12 Guilleminault, C., van den Hoed, J., Mitler, M.M. (1978) Clinical

overview of the sleep apnea syndromes, in *Sleep Apnea Syndromes* (eds C. Guilleminault, W.C. Dement), pp 1–12. New York: Liss.

13 Sullivan, C.E., Issa, F.G., Berthon-Jones, M., Eves, L. (1981) Reversal of obstructive sleep apnoea by continuous positive airway pressure applied through the nares. *Lancet*, **1**, 862–5.

14 Shapiro, C.M., Catterall, J.R., Oswald, I., Flenley, D.C. (1981) Where are the British sleep apnoea patients? *Lancet*, **2**, 523.

15 Gould, G.A., Whyte, K.F., Rhind, G.B., Airlie, M.A., Catterall, J.R., Shapiro, C.M. *et al.* (1988) The sleep hypopnea syndrome. *Am. Rev. Respir. Dis.*, **137**, 895–8.

16 American Sleep Disorders Association (ASDA). (1999) Sleep-related breathing disorders in adults: recommendations for syndrome definition and measurement techniques in clinical research. The Report of an American Academy of Sleep Medicine Task Force. *Sleep*, **22**, 667–89.

17 Guilleminault, C., Stoohs, R., Clerk, A., Cetel, M., Maistros, P. (1993) A cause of excessive daytime sleepiness. The upper airway resistance syndrome. *Chest*, **104**, 781–7.

18 Guilleminault, C., Stoohs, R., Shiomi, T., Kushida, C., Schnittger, I. (1996) Upper airway resistance syndrome, nocturnal blood pressure monitoring, and borderline hypertension. *Chest*, **109**, 901–8.

19 Douglas, N.J. (2000) Upper airway resistance syndrome is not a distinct syndrome. *Am. J. Respir. Crit. Care Med.*, **161**, 1413–15.

20 Stradling, J.R., Crosby, J.H. (1991) Predictors and prevalence of obstructive sleep apnoea and snoring in 1001 middle aged men. *Thorax*, 1991, **46**, 85–90.

21 Young, T., Palta, M., Dempsey, J., Skatrud, J., Weber, S., Badr, S. (1993) The occurrence of sleep-disordered breathing among middle-aged adults. *N. Engl. J. Med.*, **328**, 1230–5.

22 Bearpark, H., Elliott, L., Grunstein, R., Cullen, S., Schneider, H., Althaus, W. *et al.* (1995). Snoring and sleep apnea. A population study in Australian men. *Am. J. Respir. Crit. Care Med.*, **151**, 1459–65.

23 Jennum, P., Sjol, A. (1992) Epidemiology of snoring and obstructive sleep apnoea in a Danish population, age 30–60. *J. Sleep Res.*, **1**: 240–4.

24 Ancoli-Israel, S., Kripke, D.F., Mason, W., Kaplan, O.J. (1985) Sleep apnea and periodic movements in an aging sample. *J. Gerontol.*, **40**, 419–25.

25 Pendlebury, S.T., Pepin, J.L., Veale, D., Levy, P. (1997) Natural evolution of moderate sleep apnoea syndrome: significant progression over a mean of 17 months. *Thorax*, **52**, 872–8.

26 Lindberg, E., Elmasry, A., Gislason, T., Janson, C., Bengtsson, H., Hetta, J. *et al.* (1999) Evolution of sleep apnea syndrome in sleepy snorers: a population-based prospective study. *Am. J. Respir. Crit. Care Med.*, **159**, 2024–7.

27 Sforza, E., Addati, G., Cirignotta, F., Lugaresi, E. (1994) Natural evolution of sleep apnoea syndrome: a five year longitudinal study. *Eur. Respir. J.*, 7, 1765–70.

28 Jalleh, R., Fitzpatrick, M.F., Mathur, R., Douglas, N.J. (1992) Do patients with the sleep apnea/hypopnea syndrome drink more alcohol? *Sleep*, **15**, 319–21.

29 Remmers, J.E., deGroot, W.J., Sauerland, E.K., Anch, A.M. (1978) Pathogenesis of upper airway occlusion during sleep. *J. Appl. Physiol.*, **44**, 931–8.

30 Mathur, R., Mortimore, I.L., Jan, M.A., Douglas, N.J. (1995) Effect of breathing, pressure and posture on palatoglossal and genioglossal tone. *Clin. Sci. (Colch)*, **89**, 441–5.

31 Mortimore, I.L., Douglas, N.J. (1996) Palatopharyngeus has respiratory activity and responds to negative pressure in sleep apnoeics. *Eur. Respir. J.*, **9**, 773–8.

32 Mortimore, I.L., Mathur, R., Douglas, N.J. (1995) Effect of posture, route of respiration, and negative pressure on palatal muscle activity in humans. *J. Appl. Physiol.*, **79**, 448–54.

33 Tangel, D.J., Mezzanotte, W.S., White, D.P. (1991) Influence of sleep on tensor palatini EMG and upper airway resistance in normal men. *J. Appl. Physiol.*, **70**, 2574–81.

34 Onal, E., Lopata, M., O'Connor, T.D. (1981) Diaphragmatic and genioglossal electromyogram responses to isocapnic hypoxia in humans. *Am. Rev. Respir. Dis.*, **124**, 215–17.

35 Basner, R.C., Simon, P.M., Schwartzstein, R.M., Weinberger, S.E., Weiss, J.W. (1989) Breathing route influences upper airway muscle activity in awake normal adults. *J. Appl. Physiol.*, **66**, 1766–71.

36 Douglas, N.J., Jan, M.A., Yildirim, N., Warren, P.M., Drummond, G.B. (1993) Effect of posture and breathing route on genioglossal electromyogram activity in normal subjects and in patients with the sleep apnea/hypopnea syndrome. *Am. Rev. Respir. Dis.*, **148**, 1341–5.

37 Yildirim, N., Fitzpatrick, M.F., Whyte, K.F., Jalleh, R., Wightman, A.J., Douglas, N.J. (1991) The effect of posture on upper airway dimensions in normal subjects and in patients with the sleep apnea/hypopnea syndrome. *Am. Rev. Respir. Dis.*, **144**, 845–7.

38 Miyamoto, K., Ozbek, M.M., Lowe, A.A., Fleetham, J.A. (1997) Effect of body position on tongue posture in awake patients with obstructive sleep apnoea. *Thorax*, **52**, 255–9.

39 Mortimore, I.L., Fiddes, P., Stephens, S., Douglas, N.J. (1999) Tongue protrusion force and fatiguability in male and female subjects. *Eur. Respir. J.*, **14**, 191–5.

40 Horner, R.L., Innes, J.A., Murphy, K., Guz, A. (1991) Evidence for

reflex upper airway dilator muscle activation by sudden negative airway pressure in man. *J. Physiol. (Lond)*, **436**, 15–29.

41 Mortimore, I.L., Douglas, N.J. (1997) Palatal muscle EMG response to negative pressure in awake sleep apneic and control subjects. *Am. J. Respir. Crit. Care Med.*, **156**, 867–73.

42 Wheatley, J.R., Tangel, D.J., Mezzanotte, W.S., White, D.P. (1993) Influence of sleep on response to negative airway pressure of tensor palatini muscle and retropalatal airway. *J. Appl. Physiol.*, **75**, 2117–24.

43 Horner, R.L., Innes, J.A., Holden, H.B., Guz, A. (1991) Afferent pathway(s) for pharyngeal dilator reflex to negative pressure in man: a study using upper airway anaesthesia. *J. Physiol. (Lond)*, **436**, 31–44.

44 Innes, J.A., Morrell, M.J., Kobayashi, I., Hamilton, R.D., Guz, A. (1995) Central and reflex neural control of genioglossus in subjects who underwent laryngectomy. *J. Appl. Physiol.*, **78**, 2180–6.

45 Fogel, R.B., Malhotra, A., Shea, S.A., Edwards, J.K., White, D.P. (2000) Reduced genioglossal activity with upper airway anesthesia in awake patients with OSA. *J. Appl. Physiol.*, **88**, 1346–54.

46 Brooks, L.J., Strohl, K.P. (1992) Size and mechanical properties of the pharynx in healthy men and women. *Am. Rev. Respir. Dis.*, **146**, 1394–7.

47 Martin, S.E., Mathur, R., Marshall, I., Douglas, N.J. (1997) The effect of age, sex, obesity and posture on upper airway size. *Eur. Respir. J.*, 10, 2087–90.

48 Whittle, A.T., Marshall, I., Mortimore, I.L, Wraith, P.K., Sellar, R.J., Douglas, N.J. (1999) Neck soft tissue and fat distribution: comparison between normal men and women by magnetic resonance imaging. *Thorax*, **54**, 323–8.

49 White, D.P., Lombard, R.M., Cadieux, R.J., Zwillich, C.W. (1985) Pharyngeal resistance in normal humans: influence of gender, age, and obesity. *J. Appl. Physiol.*, **58**, 365–71.

50 Burger, C.D., Stanson, A.W., Daniels, B.K., Sheedy, P.F., Shepard, J.W. (1992) Fast-CT evaluation of the effect of lung volume on upper airway size and function in normal men. *Am. Rev. Respir. Dis.*, **146**, 335–9.

51 Tangel, D.J., Mezzanotte, W.S., White, D.P. (1995) Influences of NREM sleep on activity of palatoglossus and levator palatini muscles in normal men. *J. Appl. Physiol.*, **78**, 689–95.

52 Tangel, D.J., Mezzanotte, W.S., Sandberg, E.J., White, D.P. (1992) Influences of NREM sleep on the activity of tonic vs. inspiratory phasic muscles in normal men. *J. Appl. Physiol.*, **73**, 1058–66.

53 Wiegand, L., Zwillich, C.W., Wiegand, D., White, D.P. (1991) Changes in upper airway muscle activation and ventilation during phasic REM sleep in normal men. *J. Appl. Physiol.*, **71**, 488–97.

54 Horner, R.L., Innes, J.A., Morrell, M.J., Shea, S.A., Guz, A. (1994) The effect of sleep on reflex genioglossus muscle activation by stimuli of negative airway pressure in humans. *J. Physiol. (Lond)*, **476**, 141–51.

55 Haponik, E.F., Smith, P.L., Bohlman, M.E., Allen, R.P., Goldman, S.M., Bleecker, E.R. (1983) Computerized tomography in obstructive sleep apnea. Correlation of airway size with physiology during sleep and wakefulness. *Am. Rev. Respir. Dis.*, **127**, 221–6.

56 Suratt, P.M., Dee, P., Atkinson, R.L., Armstrong, P., Wilhoit, S.C. (1983) Fluoroscopic and computed tomographic features of the pharyngeal airway in obstructive sleep apnea. *Am. Rev. Respir. Dis.*, **127**, 487–92.

57 Stauffer, J.L., Zwillich, C.W., Cadieux, R.J., Bixler, E.O., Kales, A., Varano, L.A. *et al.* (1987) Pharyngeal size and resistance in obstructive sleep apnea. *Am. Rev. Respir. Dis.*, **136**, 623–7.

58 Rivlin, J., Hoffstein, V., Kalbfleisch, J., McNicholas, W., Zamel, N., Bryan, A.C. (1984) Upper airway morphology in patients with idiopathic obstructive sleep apnea. *Am. Rev. Respir. Dis.*, **129**, 355–60.

59 Martin, S.E., Marshall, I., Douglas, N.J. (1995) The effect of posture on airway caliber with the sleep-apnea/hypopnea syndrome. *Am. J. Respir. Crit. Care Med.*, **152**, 721–4.

60 Rodenstein, D.O., Dooms, G., Thomas, Y., Liistro, G., Stanescu, D.C., Culee, C. *et al.* (1990) Pharyngeal shape and dimensions in healthy subjects, snorers, and patients with obstructive sleep apnoea. *Thorax*, **45**, 722–7.

61 Schwab, R.J., Gefter, W.B., Hoffman, E.A., Gupta, K.B., Pack, A.I. (1993) Dynamic upper airway imaging during awake respiration in normal subjects and patients with sleep disordered breathing. *Am. Rev. Respir. Dis.*, **148**, 1385–400.

62 Mayer, P., Pepin, J.L., Bettega, G., Veale, D., Ferretti, G., Deschaux, C. *et al.* (1996) Relationship between body mass index, age and upper airway measurements in snorers and sleep apnoea patients. *Eur. Respir. J.*, **9**, 1801–9.

63 Horner, R.L., Mohiaddin, R.H., Lowell, D.G., Shea, S.A., Burman, E.D., Longmore, D.B. *et al.* (1989) Sites and sizes of fat deposits around the pharynx in obese patients with obstructive sleep apnoea and weight matched controls. *Eur. Respir. J.*, **2**, 613–22.

64 Shelton, K.E., Woodson, H., Gay, S., Suratt, P.M. (1993) Pharyngeal fat in obstructive sleep apnea. *Am. Rev. Respir. Dis.*, **148**, 462–6.

65 Mortimore, I.L., Marshall, I., Wraith, P.K., Sellar, R.J., Douglas, N.J. (1998) Neck and total body fat deposition in nonobese and obese patients with sleep apnea compared with that in control subjects. *Am. J. Respir. Crit. Care Med.*, **157**, 280–3.

66 Jamieson, A., Guilleminault, C., Partinen, M., Quera-Salva, M.A. (1986) Obstructive sleep apneic patients have craniomandibular abnormalities. *Sleep*, **9**, 469–77.

67 Ferguson, K.A., Ono, T., Lowe, A.A., Ryan, C.F., Fleetham, J.A. (1995) The relationship between obesity and craniofacial structure in obstructive sleep apnea. *Chest*, **108**, 375–81.

68 Kushida, C.A., Efron, B., Guilleminault, C. (1997) A predictive morphometric model for the obstructive sleep apnea syndrome. *Ann. Intern. Med.*, **127**, 581–7.

69 Mathur, R., Douglas, N.J. (1995) Family studies in patients with the sleep apnea-hypopnea syndrome. *Ann. Intern. Med.*, **122**, 174–8.

70 Ryan, C.F., Lowe, A.A., Li, D., Fleetham, J.A. (1991) Magnetic resonance imaging of the upper airway in obstructive sleep apnea before and after chronic nasal continuous positive airway pressure therapy. *Am. Rev. Respir. Dis.*, **144**, 939–44.

71 Mortimore, I.L., Kochhar, P., Douglas, N.J. (1996) Effect of chronic continuous positive airway pressure (CPAP) therapy on upper airway size in patients with sleep apnoea/hypopnoea syndrome. *Thorax*, **51**, 190–2.

72 Stauffer, J.L., Buick, M.K., Bixler, E.O., Sharkey, F.E., Abt, A.B., Manders, E.K. *et al.* (1989) Morphology of the uvula in obstructive sleep apnea. *Am. Rev. Respir. Dis.*, **140**, 724–8.

73 Riley, R., Guilleminault, C., Herran, J., Powell, N. (1983) Cephalometric analyses and flow-volume loops in obstructive sleep apnea patients. *Sleep*, **6**, 303–11.

74 Shelton, K.E., Gay, S.B., Hollowell, D.E., Woodson, H., Suratt, P.M. (1993) Mandible enclosure of upper airway and weight in obstructive sleep apnea. *Am. Rev. Respir. Dis.*, **148**, 195–200.

75 Series, F.J., Simoneau, S.A., St. Pierre, S., Marc, I. (1996) Characteristics of the genioglossus and musculus uvulae in sleep apnea hypopnea syndrome and in snorers. *Am. J. Respir. Crit. Care Med.*, **153**, 1870–4.

76 Mezzanotte, W.S., Tangel, D.J., White, D.P. (1992) Waking genioglossal electromyogram in sleep apnea patients versus normal controls (a neuromuscular compensatory mechanism). *J. Clin. Invest.*, **89**, 1571–9.

77 Suratt, P.M., McTier, R.F., Wilhoit, S.C. (1988) Upper airway muscle activation is augmented in patients with obstructive sleep apnea compared with that in normal subjects. *Am. Rev. Respir. Dis.*, **137**, 889–94.

78 Carrera, M., Barbe, F., Sauleda, J., Tomas, M., Gomez, C., Agusti, A.G. (1999) Patients with obstructive sleep apnea exhibit genioglossus dysfunction that is normalized after treatment with continuous positive airway pressure. *Am. J. Respir. Crit. Care Med.*, **159**, 1960–6.

79 Fogel, R.B., Malhotra, A., Pillar, G., Pittman, S., Edwards, J.K., Robinson, M. *et al.* (2000) The effects of surgically induced weight loss on sleep disordered breathing and pharyngeal muscle function. *Sleep,* **23** (Suppl. 2), A41.

80 Friberg, D. (1999) Heavy snorer's disease: a progressive local neuropathy. *Acta Otolaryngol.,* **119**, 925–33.

81 Findley, L.J., Wilhoit, S.C., Suratt, P.M. (1985) Apnea duration and hypoxemia during REM sleep in patients with obstructive sleep apnea. *Chest,* **87**, 432–6.

82 Issa, F.G., Sullivan, C.E. (1984) Upper airway closing pressures in obstructive sleep apnea. *J. Appl. Physiol.,* **57**, 520–7.

83 Gleadhill, I.C., Schwartz, A.R., Schubert, N., Wise, R.A., Permutt, S., Smith, P.L. (1991) Upper airway collapsibility in snorers and in patients with obstructive hypopnea and apnea. *Am. Rev. Respir. Dis.,* **143**, 1300–3.

84 Schwartz, A.R., Gold, A.R., Schubert, N., Stryzak, A., Wise, R.A., Permutt, S. *et al.* (1991) Effect of weight loss on upper airway collapsibility in obstructive sleep apnea. *Am. Rev. Respir. Dis.,* **144**, 494–8.

85 Series, F., Roy, N., Marc, I. (1994) Effects of sleep deprivation and sleep fragmentation on upper airway collapsibility in normal subjects. *Am. J. Respir. Crit. Care Med.,* **150**, 481–5.

86 Meurice, J.C., Marc, I., Carrier, G., Series, F. (1996) Effects of mouth opening on upper airway collapsibility in normal sleeping subjects. *Am. J. Respir. Crit. Care Med., 153*, 255–9.

87 Morrison, D.L., Launois, S.H., Isono, S., Feroah, T.R., Whitelaw, W.A., Remmers, J.E. (1993) Pharyngeal narrowing and closing pressures in patients with obstructive sleep apnea. *Am. Rev. Respir. Dis.,* **148**, 606–11.

88 Hudgel, D.W. (1986) Variable site of airway narrowing among obstructive sleep apnea patients. *J. Appl. Physiol.,* **61**, 1403–9.

89 Chaban, R., Cole, P., Hoffstein, V. (1988) Site of upper airway obstruction in patients with idiopathic obstructive sleep apnea. *Laryngoscope,* **98**, 641–7.

90 Douglas, N. (1997) Surgical treatment for obstructive sleep apnoea. *Sleep Medicine Reviews,* **1**, 77–86.

91 Smith, P.L., Haponik, E.F., Bleecker, E.R. (1984) The effects of oxygen in patients with sleep apnea. *Am. Rev. Respir. Dis.,* **130**, 958–63.

92 Douglas, N.J., White, D.P., Weil, J.V., Pickett, C.K., Zwillich, C.W. (1982) Hypercapnic ventilatory response in sleeping adults. *Am. Rev. Respir. Dis.,* **126**, 758–62.

93 Gleeson, K., Zwillich, C.W., White, D.P. (1990) The influence of increasing ventilatory effort on arousal from sleep. *Am. Rev. Respir. Dis.,* **142**, 295–300.

94 Vincken, W., Guilleminault, C., Silvestri, L., Cosio, M., Grassino, A.

(1987) Inspiratory muscle activity as a trigger causing the airways to open in obstructive sleep apnea. *Am. Rev. Respir. Dis.*, **135**, 372–7.

95 Douglas, N.J., Polo, O. (1994) Pathogenesis of obstructive sleep apnoea/hypopnoea syndrome. *Lancet*, **344**, 653–5.

96 Engleman, H., Joffe, D. (1999) Neuropsychological function in obstructive sleep apnoea. *Sleep Medicine Reviews*, **3**, 59–78.

97 Davies, R.J., Crosby, J., Vardi-Visy, K., Clarke, M., Stradling, J.R. (1994) Non-invasive beat to beat arterial blood pressure during non-REM sleep in obstructive sleep apnoea and snoring. *Thorax*, **49**, 335–9.

98 Martin, S.E., Engleman, H.M., Deary, I.J., Douglas, N.J. (1996) The effect of sleep fragmentation on daytime function. *Am. J. Respir. Crit. Care Med.*, **153**, 1328–32.

99 Kingshott, R.N., Engleman, H.M., Deary, I.J., Douglas, N.J. (1998) Does arousal frequency predict daytime function? *Eur. Respir. J.*, **12**, 1264–70.

100 Kingshott, R.N., Vennelle, M., Hoy, C.J., Engleman, H.M., Deary, I.J., Douglas, N.J. (2000) Predictors of improvements in daytime function outcomes with CPAP therapy. *Am. J. Respir. Crit. Care Med.*, **161**, 866–71.

101 Bennett, L.S., Stradling, J.R., Davies, R.J. (1997) A behavioural test to assess daytime sleepiness in obstructive sleep apnoea. *J. Sleep. Res.*, **6**, 142–5.

102 Martin, S.E., Wraith, P.K., Deary, I.J., Douglas, N.J. (1997) The effect of nonvisible sleep fragmentation on daytime function. *Am. J. Respir. Crit. Care Med.*, **155**, 1596–601.

103 Bennett, L.S., Langford, B.A., Stradling, J.R., Davies, R.J.O. (1998) Sleep fragmentation indices as predictors of daytime sleepiness and nCPAP response in obstructive sleep apnea [In Process Citation]. *Am. J. Respir. Crit. Care Med.*, **158**, 778–86.

104 Ali, N.J., Davies, R.J., Fleetham, J.A., Stradling, J.R. (1991) Periodic movements of the legs during sleep associated with rises in systemic blood pressure. *Sleep*, **14**, 163–5.

105 Bristow, J.D., Honour, A.J., Pickering, T.G., Sleight, P. (1969) Cardiovascular and respiratory changes during sleep in normal and hypertensive subjects. *Cardiovasc. Res.*, **3**, 476–85.

106 Somers, V.K., Dyken, M.E., Mark, A.L., Abboud, F.M. (1993) Sympathetic-nerve activity during sleep in normal subjects. *N. Engl. J. Med.*, **328**, 303–7.

107 Sforza, E., Krieger, J., Petiau, C. (1998) Nocturnal evolution of respiratory effort in obstructive sleep apnoea syndrome: influence on arousal threshold. *Eur. Respir. J.*, **12**, 1257–63.

108 McEvoy, R.D., Sharp, D.J., Thornton, A.T. (1986) The effects of

posture on obstructive sleep apnea. *Am. Rev. Respir. Dis.*, **133**, 662–6.

109 Redline, S., Tishler, P.V., Tosteson, T.D., Williamson, J., Kump, K., Browner, I. *et al.* (1995) The familial aggregation of obstructive sleep apnea. *Am. J. Respir. Crit. Care Med.*, **151**, 682–7.

110 Stunkard, A.J., Sorensen, T.I., Hanis, C., Teasdale, T.W., Chakraborty, R., Schull, W.J. *et al.* (1986) An adoption study of human obesity. *N. Engl. J. Med.*, 314, 193–8.

111 Engleman, H.M., Hirst, W.S., Douglas, N.J. (1997) Under reporting of sleepiness and driving impairment in patients with sleep apnoea/hypopnoea syndrome. *J. Sleep. Res.*, **6**, 272–5.

112 British Sleep Foundation. (2000) Sleepiness when driving. (www.britishsleepfoundation.org.uk).

113 Maycock, G. (1996) Sleepiness and driving: the experience of UK car drivers. *J. Sleep Res.*, 5, 229–37.

114 Teran-Santos, J., Jimenez-Gomez, A., Cordero-Guevara, J. (1999) The association between sleep apnea and the risk of traffic accidents. Cooperative Group Burgos-Santander. *N. Engl. J. Med.*, **340**, 847–51.

115 Young, T., Blustein, J., Finn, L., Palta, M. (1997) Sleep-disordered breathing and motor vehicle accidents in a population-based sample of employed adults. *Sleep*, **20**, 608–13.

116 Horstmann, S., Hess, C.W., Bassetti, C., Gugger, M., Mathis, J. (2000) Sleepiness-related accidents in sleep apnea patients. *Sleep*, **23**, 383–9.

117 Barbe, F., Pericas, J., Munoz, A., Findley, L., Anto, J.M., Agusti, A.G. (1998) Automobile accidents in patients with sleep apnea syndrome. An epidemiological and mechanistic study. *Am. J. Respir. Crit. Care Med.*, **158**, 18–22.

118 Findley, L.J., Unverzagt, M.E., Suratt, P.M. (1998) Automobile accidents involving patients with obstructive sleep apnea. *Am. Rev. Respir. Dis.*, **138**, 337–40.

119 George, C.F., Smiley, A. (1999) Sleep apnea and automobile crashes. *Sleep*, **22**, 790–5.

120 Findley, L.J., Fabrizio, M.J., Knight, H., Norcross, B.B., LaForte, A.J., Suratt, P.M. (1989) Driving simulator performance in patients with sleep apnea. *Am. Rev. Respir. Dis.*, 140, 529–30.

121 Findley, L., Unverzagt, M., Guchu, R., Fabrizio, M., Buckner, J., Suratt, P. (1995) Vigilance and automobile accidents in patients with sleep apnea or narcolepsy. *Chest*, **108**, 619–24.

122 George, C.F., Boudreau, A.C., Smiley, A. (1996) Comparison of simulated driving performance in narcolepsy and sleep apnea patients. *Sleep*, **19**, 711–17.

123 George, C.F., Boudreau, A.C., Smiley, A. (1996) Simulated driving

performance in patients with obstructive sleep apnea. *Am. J. Respir. Crit. Care Med.*, **154**, 175–81.

124 Risser, M.R., Ware, J.C., Freeman, F.G. (2000) Driving simulation with EEG monitoring in normal and obstructive sleep apnea patients. *Sleep*, **23**, 393–8.

125 George, C.F., Boudreau, A.C., Smiley, A. (1997) Effects of nasal CPAP on simulated driving performance in patients with obstructive sleep apnoea. *Thorax*, **52**, 648–53.

126 Hack, M., Davies, R.J., Mullins, R., Choi, S.J., Ramdassingh-Dow, S., Jenkinson, C. *et al.* (2000) Randomised prospective parallel trial of therapeutic versus subtherapeutic nasal continuous positive airway pressure on simulated steering performance in patients with obstructive sleep apnoea. *Thorax*, **55**, 224–31.

127 Krieger, J., Meslier, N., Lebrun, T., Levy, P., Phillip-Joet, F., Sailly, J.C. *et al.* (1997) Accidents in obstructive sleep apnea patients treated with nasal continuous positive airway pressure: a prospective study. The Working Group ANTADIR, Paris and CRESGE, Lille, France. Association Nationale de Traitement a Domicile des Insuffisants Respiratoires. *Chest*, **112**, 1561–6.

128 George, C.F. (2001) Reduction in motor vehicle collisions following treatment of sleep apnoea with nasal CPAP. *Thorax*, **56**, 508–12.

129 Ulfberg, J., Carter, N., Edling, C. (2000) Sleep-disordered breathing and occupational accidents. *Scand. J. Work Environ. Health*, **26**, 237–42.

130 Bedard, M.A., Montplaisir, J., Richer, F., Rouleau, I., Malo, J. (1991) Obstructive sleep apnea syndrome: pathogenesis of neuropsychological deficits. *J. Clin. Exp. Neuropsychol.*, **13**, 950–64.

131 Naegele, B., Thouvard, V., Pepin, J.L., Levy, P., Bonnet, C., Perret, J.E. *et al.* (1995) Deficits of cognitive executive functions in patients with sleep apnea syndrome. *Sleep*, **18**, 43–52.

132 Cheshire, K., Engleman, H., Deary, I., Shapiro, C., Douglas, N.J. (1992) Factors impairing daytime performance in patients with sleep apnea/hypopnea syndrome. *Arch. Intern. Med.*, **152**, 538–41.

133 Engleman, H.M., Cheshire, K.E., Deary, I.J., Douglas, N.J. (1993) Daytime sleepiness, cognitive performance and mood after continuous positive airway pressure for the sleep apnoea/hypopnoea syndrome. *Thorax*, **48**, 911–14.

134 Engleman, H.M., Kingshott, R.N., Wraith, P.K., Mackay, T.W., Deary, I.J., Douglas, N.J. (1999) Randomized placebo-controlled crossover trial of continuous positive airway pressure for mild sleep apnea/hypopnea syndrome. *Am. J. Respir. Crit. Care Med.*, **159**, 461–7.

135 Douglas, N.J. (1998) Systematic review of the efficacy of nasal CPAP. *Thorax*, **53**, 414–15.

136 Norton, P.G., Dunn, E.V. (1985) Snoring as a risk factor for disease: an epidemiological survey. *BMJ*, **291**, 630–2.

137 Koskenvuo, M., Kaprio, J., Partinen, M., Langinvainio, H., Sarna, S., Heikkila, K. (1985) Snoring as a risk factor for hypertension and angina pectoris. *Lancet*, **1**, 893–6.

138 Olson, L.G., King, M.T., Hensley, M.J., Saunders, N.A. (1995) A community study of snoring and sleep-disordered breathing. Health outcomes. *Am. J. Respir. Crit. Care Med.* **152**, 717–20.

139 Motta, J., Guilleminault, C., Schroeder, J.S., Dement, W.C. (1978) Tracheostomy and hemodynamic changes in sleep-inducing apnea. *Ann. Intern. Med.*, **89**, 454–8.

140 Carlson, J.T., Hedner, J.A., Ejnell, H., Peterson, L.E. (1994) High prevalence of hypertension in sleep apnea patients independent of obesity. *Am. J. Respir. Crit. Care Med.* **150**, 72–7.

141 Worsnop, C.J., Naughton, M.T., Barter, C.E., Morgan, T.O., Anderson, A.I., Pierce, R.J. (1998) The prevalence of obstructive sleep apnea in hypertensives. *Am. J. Respir. Crit. Care Med.*, **157**, 111–15.

142 Lavie, P., Ben Yosef, R., Rubin, A.E. (1984) Prevalence of sleep apnea syndrome among patients with essential hypertension. *Am. Heart J.*, **108**, 373–6.

143 Fletcher, E.C., DeBehnke, R.D., Lovoi, M.S., Gorin, A.B. (1985) Undiagnosed sleep apnea in patients with essential hypertension. *Ann. Intern. Med.*, **103**, 190–5.

144 Kales, A., Bixler, E.O., Cadieux, R.J., Schneck, D.W., Shaw, L.C., Locke, T.W. *et al.* (1984) Sleep apnoea in a hypertensive population. *Lancet*, **2**, 1005–8.

145 Brooks, D., Horner, R.L., Kozar, L.F., Render-Teixeira, C.L., Phillipson, E.A. (1997) Obstructive sleep apnea as a cause of systemic hypertension. Evidence from a canine model. *J. Clin. Invest.*, **99**, 106–9.

146 Brooks, D., Horner, R.L., Kimoff, R.J., Kozar, L.F., Render-Teixeira, C.L., Phillipson, E.A. (1997) Effect of obstructive sleep apnea versus sleep fragmentation on responses to airway occlusion. *Am. J. Respir. Crit. Care Med.*, **155**, 1609–17.

147 Fletcher, E.C., Lesske, J., Qian, W., Miller, C.C., Unger, T. (1992) Repetitive, episodic hypoxia causes diurnal elevation of blood pressure in rats. *Hypertension*, **19**, 555–61.

148 Lesske, J., Fletcher, E.C., Bao, G., Unger, T. (1997) Hypertension caused by chronic intermittent hypoxia – influence of chemoreceptors and sympathetic nervous system. *J. Hypertens.*, **15**, 1593–603.

149 Bao, G., Metreveli, N., Fletcher, E.C. (1999) Acute and chronic blood pressure response to recurrent acoustic arousal in rats. *Am. J. Hypertens.*, **12**, 504–10.

150 Hla, K.M., Young, T.B., Bidwell, T., Palta, M., Skatrud, J.B., Dempsey,

J. (1994) Sleep apnea and hypertension. A population-based study. *Ann. Intern. Med.*, **120**, 382–8.

151 Peppard, P.E., Young, T., Palta, M., Skatrud, J. (2000) Prospective study of the association between sleep-disordered breathing and hypertension. *N. Engl. J. Med.*, **342**, 1378–84.

152 Nieto, F.J., Young, T.B., Lind, B.K., Shahar, E., Samet, J.M., Redline, S. *et al.* (2000) Association of sleep-disordered breathing, sleep apnea, and hypertension in a large community-based study. Sleep Heart Health Study. *JAMA*, **283**, 1829–36.

153 Young, T., Peppard, P., Palta, M., Hla, K.M., Finn, L., Morgan, B. *et al.* (1997) Population-based study of sleep-disordered breathing as a risk factor for hypertension. *Arch. Intern. Med.*, **157**, 1746–52.

154 Bixler, E.O., Vgontzas, A.N., Lin, H.M., Ten Have, T., Leiby, B.E., Vela-Bueno, A. *et al.* (2000) Association of hypertension and sleep-disordered breathing. *Arch. Intern. Med.*, **160**, 2289–95.

155 Lavie, P., Herer, P., Hoffstein, V. (2000) Obstructive sleep apnoea syndrome as a risk factor for hypertension: population study. *BMJ*, **320**, 479–82.

156 Grunstein, R.R., Ho, K.Y., Sullivan, C.E. (1991) Sleep apnea in acromegaly. *Ann. Intern. Med.*, **115**, 527–32.

157 Grote, L., Ploch, T., Heitmann, J., Knaack, L., Penzel, T., Peter, J.H. (1999) Sleep-related breathing disorder is an independent risk factor for systemic hypertension. *Am. J. Respir. Crit. Care Med.*, **160**, 1875–82.

158 Davies, C.W., Crosby, J.H., Mullins, R.L., Barbour, C., Davies, R.J., Stradling, J.R. (2000) Case-control study of 24 hour ambulatory blood pressure in patients with obstructive sleep apnoea and normal matched control subjects. *Thorax*, **55**, 736–40.

159 Faccenda, J.F., Mackay, T.W., Boon, N.A., Douglas, N.J. (2001) Randomized placebo-controlled trial of continuous positive airway pressure on blood pressure in the sleep apnea–hypopnea syndrome. *Am. J. Respir. Crit. Care Med.*, **163**, 344–8.

160 MacMahon, S., Peto, R., Cutler, J., Collins, R., Sorlie, P., Neaton, J. *et al.* (1990) Blood pressure, stroke, and coronary heart disease. Part 1, Prolonged differences in blood pressure: prospective observational studies corrected for the regression dilution bias. *Lancet*, **335**, 765–74.

161 Collins, R., Peto, R., MacMahon, S., Hebert, P., Fiebach, N.H., Eberlein, K.A. *et al.* (1990) Blood pressure, stroke, and coronary heart disease. Part 2, Short-term reductions in blood pressure: overview of randomised drug trials in their epidemiological context. *Lancet*, **335**, 827–38.

162 Hung, J., Whitford, E.G., Parsons, R.W., Hillman, D.R. (1990) Association of sleep apnoea with myocardial infarction in men. *Lancet*, **336**, 261–4.

163 Lanfranchi, P.A., Braghiroli, A., Bosimini, E., Mazzuero, G., Colombo, R., Donner, C.F. *et al.* (1999) Prognostic value of nocturnal Cheyne–Stokes respiration in chronic heart failure. *Circulation*, **99**, 1435–40.

164 Partinen, M., Jamieson, A., Guilleminault, C. (1988) Long-term outcome for obstructive sleep apnea syndrome patients. Mortality. *Chest*, **94**, 1200–4.

165 Partinen, M., Guilleminault, C. (1990) Daytime sleepiness and vascular morbidity at seven-year follow-up in obstructive sleep apnea patients. *Chest*, **97**, 27–32.

166 Shahar, E., Whitney, C.W., Redline, S., Lee, E.T., Newman, A.B., Javier, N.F. *et al.* (2001) Sleep-disordered breathing and cardiovascular disease. Cross-sectional results of the sleep heart health study. *Am. J. Respir. Crit. Care Med.*, **163**, 19–25.

167 Dyken, M.E., Somers, V.K., Yamada, T., Ren, Z.Y., Zimmerman, M.B. (1996) Investigating the relationship between stroke and obstructive sleep apnea. *Stroke*, **27**, 401–7.

168 Bassetti, C., Aldrich, M.S., Chervin, R.D., Quint, D. (1996) Sleep apnea in patients with transient ischemic attack and stroke: a prospective study of 59 patients. *Neurology*, **47**, 1167–73.

169 Good, D.C., Henkle, J.Q., Gelber, D., Welsh, J., Verhulst, S. (1996) Sleep-disordered breathing and poor functional outcome after stroke. *Stroke*, **27**, 252–9.

170 Koskenvuo, M., Kaprio, J., Telakivi, T., Partinen, M., Heikkila, K., Sarna, S. (1987) Snoring as a risk factor for ischaemic heart disease and stroke in men. *BMJ*, **294**, 16–19.

171 Palomaki, H., Partinen, M., Erkinjuntti, T., Kaste, M. (1992) Snoring, sleep apnea syndrome, and stroke. *Neurology*, **42**, 75–81; discussion 82.

172 Palomaki, H., Partinen, M., Juvela, S., Kaste, M. (1989) Snoring as a risk factor for sleep-related brain infarction. *Stroke*, **20**, 1311–15.

173 Spriggs, D.A., French, J.M., Murdy, J.M., Curless, R.H., Bates, D., James, O.F. (1992) Snoring increases the risk of stroke and adversely affects prognosis. *Q. J. Med.*, **83**, 555–62.

174 Bradley, T.D., Rutherford, R., Grossman, R.F., Lue, F., Zamel, N., Moldofsky, H. *et al.* (1985) Role of daytime hypoxemia in the pathogenesis of right heart failure in the obstructive sleep apnea syndrome. *Am. Rev. Respir. Dis.*, **131**, 835–9.

175 Whyte, K.F., Douglas, N.J. (1991) Peripheral edema in the sleep apnea/hypopnea syndrome. *Sleep*, **14**, 354–6.

176 Bradley, T.D., Rutherford, R., Lue, F., Moldofsky, H., Grossman, R.F., Zamel, N. *et al.* (1986) Role of diffuse airway obstruction in the hypercapnia of obstructive sleep apnea. *Am. Rev. Respir. Dis.*, **134**, 920–4.

177 Fletcher, E.C., Schaaf, J.W., Miller, J., Fletcher, J.G. (1987) Long-term cardiopulmonary sequelae in patients with sleep apnea and chronic lung disease. *Am. Rev. Respir. Dis.*, **135**, 525–33.

178 Berthon-Jones, M., Sullivan, C.E. (1987) Time course of change in ventilatory response to CO_2 with long-term CPAP therapy for obstructive sleep apnea. *Am. Rev. Respir. Dis.*, **135**, 144–7.

179 Goldman, J.M., Ireland, R.M., Berthon-Jones, M., Grunstein, R.R., Sullivan, C.E., Biggs, J.C. (1991) Erythropoietin concentrations in obstructive sleep apnoea. *Thorax*, **46**, 25–7.

180 Pokala, P., Llanera, M., Sherwood, J., Scharf, S., Steinberg, H. (1995) Erythropoietin response in subjects with obstructive sleep apnea. *Am. J. Respir. Crit. Care Med.*, **151**, 1862–5.

181 Hiremath, A.S., Hillman, D.R., James, A.L., Noffsinger, W.J., Platt, P.R., Singer, S.L. (1998) Relationship between difficult tracheal intubation and obstructive sleep apnoea. *Br. J. Anaesth.*, **80**, 606–11.

182 Kahn, A., Groswasser, J., Rebuffat, E., Sottiaux, M., Blum, D., Foerster, M. *et al.* (1992) Sleep and cardiorespiratory characteristics of infant victims of sudden death: a prospective case-control study. *Sleep*, **15**, 287–92.

183 Mathur, R., Douglas, N.J. (1994) Relation between sudden infant death syndrome and adult sleep apnoea/hypopnoea syndrome. *Lancet*, **344**, 819–20.

184 Tishler, P.V., Redline, S., Ferrette, V., Hans, M.G., Altose, M.D. (1996) The association of sudden unexpected infant death with obstructive sleep apnea. *Am. J. Respir. Crit. Care Med.*, **153**, 1857–63.

185 Guilleminault, C., Heldt, G., Powell, N., Riley, R. (1986) Small upper airway in near-miss sudden infant death syndrome infants and their families. *Lancet*, **1**, 402–7.

186 Rees, K., Wright, A., Keeling, J.W., Douglas, N.J. (1998) Facial structure in the sudden infant death syndrome: case- control study. *BMJ*, **317**, 179–80.

187 Whyte, K.F., Allen, M.B., Jeffrey, A.A., Gould, G.A., Douglas, N.J. (1989) Clinical features of the sleep apnoea/hypopnoea syndrome. *Q. J. Med.*, **72**, 659–66.

188 Johns, M.W. (1991) A new method for measuring daytime sleepiness: the Epworth sleepiness scale. *Sleep*, **14**, 540–5.

189 Parkes, J.D., Chen, S.Y., Clift, S.J., Dahlitz, M.J., Dunn, G. (1998) The clinical diagnosis of the narcoleptic syndrome. *J. Sleep. Res.*, **7**, 41–52.

190 Kingshott, R.N., Sime, P.J., Engleman, H.M., Douglas, N.J. (1995) Self assessment of daytime sleepiness: patient versus partner. *Thorax*, **50**, 994–5.

191 Engleman, H.M., Martin, S.E., Deary, I.J., Douglas, N.J. (1994)

Effect of continuous positive airway pressure treatment on daytime function in sleep apnoea/hypopnoea syndrome. *Lancet*, **343**, 572–5.

192 Warley, A.R., Stradling, J.R. (1988) Abnormal diurnal variation in salt and water excretion in patients with obstructive sleep apnoea. *Clin. Sci.*, **74**, 183–5.

193 Lin, C.C., Tsan, K.W., Lin, C.Y. (1993) Plasma levels of atrial natriuretic factor in moderate to severe obstructive sleep apnea syndrome. *Sleep*, **16**, 37–9.

194 Poceta, J.S., Dalessio, D.J. (1995) Identification and treatment of sleep apnea in patients with chronic headache. *Headache*, **35**, 586–9.

195 Hill, A.T., Edenborough, F.P., Cayton, R.M., Stableforth, D.E. (1998) Long-term nasal intermittent positive pressure ventilation in patients with cystic fibrosis and hypercapnic respiratory failure (1991–1996). *Respir. Med.*, **92**, 5236.

196 Crocker, B.D., Olson, L.G., Saunders, N.A., Hensley, M.J., McKeon, J.L., Allen, K.M. *et al.* (1990) Estimation of the probability of disturbed breathing during sleep before a sleep study. *Am. Rev. Respir. Dis.*, **142**, 14–8.

197 Flemons, W.W., Whitelaw, W.A., Brant, R., Remmers, J.E. (1994) Likelihood ratios for a sleep apnea clinical prediction rule. *Am. J. Respir. Crit. Care Med.*, **150**, 1279–85.

198 Kump, K., Whalen, C., Tishler, P.V., Browner, I., Ferrette, V., Strohl, K.P. *et al.* (1994) Assessment of the validity and utility of a sleep-symptom questionnaire. *Am. J. Respir. Crit. Care Med.*, **150**, 735–41.

199 Hoffstein, V., Mateika, S. (1992) Differences in abdominal and neck circumferences in patients with and without obstructive sleep apnoea. *Eur. Respir. J.*, **5**, 377–81.

200 Hoffstein, V., Szalai, J.P. (1993) Predictive value of clinical features in diagnosing obstructive sleep apnea. *Sleep*, **16**, 118–22.

201 Guilleminault, C., Cummiskey, J. (1982) Progressive improvement of apnea index and ventilatory response to CO_2 after tracheostomy in obstructive sleep apnea syndrome. *Am. Rev. Respir. Dis.*, **126**, 14–20.

202 Grunstein, R.R., Sullivan, C.E. (1988) Sleep apnea and hypothyroidism: mechanisms and management. *Am. J. Med.*, **85**, 775–9.

203 Cistulli, P.A., Sullivan, C.E. (1993) Sleep-disordered breathing in Marfan's syndrome. *Am. Rev. Respir. Dis.*, **147**, 645–8.

204 Viner, S., Szalai, J.P., Hoffstein, V. (1991) Are history and physical examination a good screening test for sleep apnea? *Ann. Intern. Med.*, **115**, 356–9.

205 Maislin, G., Pack, A.I., Kribbs, N.B., Smith, P.L., Schwartz, A.R., Kline, L.R. *et al.* (1995) A survey screen for prediction of apnea. *Sleep*, **18**, 158–66.

206 Katz, I., Zamel, N., Slutsky, A.S., Rebuck, A.S., Hoffstein, V. (1990)

An evaluation of flow-volume curves as a screening test for obstructive sleep apnea. *Chest*, **98**, 337–40.

207 Skjodt, N.M., Atkar, R., Easton, P.A. (1999) Screening for hypothyroidism in sleep apnea. *Am. J. Respir. Crit. Care Med.*, **160**, 732–5.

208 Lin, C.C., Tsan, K.W., Chen, P.J. (1992) The relationship between sleep apnea syndrome and hypothyroidism. *Chest*, **102**, 1663–7.

209 Winkelman, J.W., Goldman, H., Piscatelli, N., Lukas, S.E., Dorsey, C.M., Cunningham, S. (1996) Are thyroid function tests necessary in patients with suspected sleep apnea? *Sleep*, **19**, 790–3.

210 Whittle, A.T., Finch, S.P., Mortimore, I.L., Mackay, T.W., Douglas, N.J. (1997) Use of home sleep studies for diagnosis of the sleep apnoea/hypopnoea syndrome. *Thorax*, **52**, 1068–73.

211 Rees, K., Wraith, P.K., Berthon-Jones, M., Douglas, N.J. (1998) Detection of apnoeas, hypopnoeas and arousals by the AutoSet in the sleep apnoea/hypopnoea syndrome. *Eur. Respir. J.*, **12**, 764–9.

212 Krieger, J., Sforza, E., Petiau, C., Weiss, T. (1998) Simplified diagnostic procedure for obstructive sleep apnoea syndrome: lower subsequent compliance with CPAP. *Eur. Respir. J.*, **12**, 776–9.

213 Montserrat, J.M., Farre, R., Ballester, E., Felez, M.A., Pasto, M., Navajas, D. (1997) Evaluation of nasal prongs for estimating nasal flow. *Am. J. Respir. Crit. Care Med.*, **155**, 211–15.

214 Ballester, E., Badia, J.R., Hernandez, L., Farre, R., Navajas, D., Montserrat, J.M. (1998) Nasal prongs in the detection of sleep-related disordered breathing in the sleep apnoea/hypopnoea syndrome. *Eur. Respir. J.*, **11**, 880–3.

215 Series, F., Marc, I. (1999) Nasal pressure recording in the diagnosis of sleep apnoea hypopnoea syndrome. *Thorax*, **54**, 506–10.

216 Guilleminault, C., Stoohs, R., Duncan, S. (1991) Snoring (I). Daytime sleepiness in regular heavy snorers. *Chest*, **99**, 40–8.

217 Davies, R.J., Vardi-Visy, K., Clarke, M., Stradling, J.R. (1993) Identification of sleep disruption and sleep disordered breathing from the systolic blood pressure profile. *Thorax*, **48**, 1242–7.

218 Norman, R.G., Ahmed, M.M., Walsleben, J.A., Rapoport, D.M. (1997) Detection of respiratory events during NPSG: nasal cannula/pressure sensor versus thermistor. *Sleep*, **20**, 1175–84.

219 Rees, K., Kingshott, R.N., Wraith, P.K., Douglas, N.J. (2000) Frequency and significance of increased upper airway resistance during sleep. *Am. J. Respir. Crit. Care Med.*, **162**, 1210–14.

220 Badia, J.R., Farre, R.O., John, K.R., Ballester, E., Hernandez, L., Rotger, M. *et al.* (1999) Clinical application of the forced oscillation technique for CPAP titration in the sleep apnea/hypopnea syndrome. *Am. J. Respir. Crit. Care Med.*, **160**, 1550–4.

221 Pitson, D.J., Stradling, J.R. (1998) Value of beat-to-beat blood pressure

249 McArdle, N., Devereux, G., Heidarnejad, H., Engleman, H.M., Mackay, T.W., Douglas, N.J. (1999) Long-term use of CPAP therapy for sleep apnea/hypopnea syndrome. *Am. J. Respir. Crit. Care Med.*, **159**, 1108–14.

250 Chervin, R.D., Theut, S., Bassetti, C., Aldrich, M.S. (1997) Compliance with nasal CPAP can be improved by simple interventions. *Sleep*, **20**, 284–9.

251 Hoy, C.J., Vennelle, M., Kingshott, R.N., Engleman, H.M., Douglas, N.J. (1999) Can intensive support improve continuous positive airway pressure use in patients with the sleep apnea/hypopnea syndrome? *Am. J. Respir. Crit. Care Med.*, **159**, 1096–100.

252 Whittle, A.T., Douglas, N.J. (2000) Does the physiological success of CPAP titration predict clinical success? *J. Sleep Res.*, **9**, 201–6.

253 Lloberes, P., Ballester, E., Montserrat, J.M., Botifoll, E., Ramirez, A., Reolid, A. *et al.* (1996) Comparison of manual and automatic CPAP titration in patients with sleep apnea/hypopnea syndrome. *Am. J. Respir. Crit. Care Med.*, **154**, 1755–8.

254 Teschler, H., Berthon-Jones, M., Thompson, A.B., Henkel, A., Henry, J., Konietzko, N. (1996) Automated continuous positive airway pressure titration for obstructive sleep apnea syndrome. *Am. J. Respir. Crit. Care Med.*, **154**, 734–40.

255 Stradling, J.R., Barbour, C., Pitson, D.J., Davies, R.J. (1997) Automatic nasal continuous positive airway pressure titration in the laboratory: patient outcomes. *Thorax*, **52**, 72–5.

256 Strollo, P.J., Sanders, M.H., Costantino, J.P., Walsh, S.K., Stiller, R.A., Atwood, C.W. (1996) Split-night studies for the diagnosis and treatment of sleep-disordered breathing. *Sleep*, **19**, S255–S259.

257 Yamashiro, Y., Kryger, M.H. (1995) CPAP titration for sleep apnea using a split-night protocol. *Chest*, **107**, 62–6.

258 Fleury, B., Rakotonanahary, D., Tehindrazanarivelo, A.D., Hausser-Hauw, C., Lebeau, B. (1994) Long-term compliance to continuous positive airway pressure therapy (nCPAP) set up during a split-night polysomnography. *Sleep*, **17**, 512–15.

259 McArdle, N., Grove, A., Devereux, G., Mackay-Brown, L., Mackay, T., Douglas, N.J. (2000) Split-night versus full-night studies for sleep apnoea/hypopnoea syndrome. *Eur. Respir. J.*, **15**, 670–5.

260 Weaver, T.E., Kribbs, N.B., Pack, A.I., Kline, L.R., Chugh, D.K., Maislin, G. *et al.* (1997) Night-to-night variability in CPAP use over the first three months of treatment. *Sleep*, **20**, 278–83.

261 Mawhinney, H., Spector, S.L., Kinsman, R.A., Siegel, S.C., Rachelefsky, G.S., Katz, R.M. *et al.* (1991) Compliance in clinical trials of two nonbronchodilator, antiasthma medications. *Ann. Allergy*, **66**, 294–9.

262 Rudd, P. (1995) Clinicians and patients with hypertension: unsettled issues about compliance. *Am. Heart J.*, **130**, 572–9.

263 Reeves-Hoche, M.K., Meck, R., Zwillich, C.W. (1994) Nasal CPAP: an objective evaluation of patient compliance. *Am. J. Respir. Crit. Care Med.*, **149**, 149–54.

264 Engleman, H.M., Martin, S.E., Douglas, N.J. (1994) Compliance with CPAP therapy in patients with the sleep apnoea/hypopnoea syndrome. *Thorax*, **49**, 263–6.

265 Rauscher, H., Formanek, D., Popp, W., Zwick, H. (1993) Self-reported vs measured compliance with nasal CPAP for obstructive sleep apnea. *Chest*, **103**, 1675–80.

266 Engleman, H.M., Martin, S.E., Kingshott, R.N., Mackay, T.W., Deary, I.J., Douglas, N.J. (1998) Randomised placebo controlled trial of daytime function after continuous positive airway pressure (CPAP) therapy for the sleep apnoea/hypopnoea syndrome. *Thorax*, **53**, 341–5.

267 Engleman, H.M., Asgari-Jirhandeh, N., McLeod, A.L., Ramsay, C.F., Deary, I.J., Douglas, N.J. (1996) Self-reported use of CPAP and benefits of CPAP therapy: a patient survey. *Chest*, **109**, 1470–6.

268 Krieger, J., Kurtz, D., Petiau, C., Sforza, E., Trautmann, D. (1996) Long-term compliance with CPAP therapy in obstructive sleep apnea patients and in snorers. *Sleep*, **19**, S136–S143.

269 Rauscher, H., Popp, W., Wanke, T., Zwick, H. (1991) Acceptance of CPAP therapy for sleep apnea. *Chest*, **100**, 1019–23.

270 Kribbs, N.B., Pack, A.I., Kline, L.R., Smith, P.L., Schwartz, A.R., Schubert, N.M. *et al.* (1993) Objective measurement of patterns of nasal CPAP use by patients with obstructive sleep apnea. *Am. Rev. Respir. Dis.*, **147**, 887–95.

271 Jarjour, N.N., Wilson, P. (1989) Pneumocephalus associated with nasal continuous positive airway pressure in a patient with sleep apnea syndrome. *Chest*, **96**, 1425–6.

272 Richards, G.N., Cistulli, P.A., Ungar, R.G., Berthon-Jones, M., Sullivan, C.E. (1996) Mouth leak with nasal continuous positive airway pressure increases nasal airway resistance. *Am. J. Respir. Crit. Care Med.*, **154**, 182–6.

273 Mortimore, I.L., Whittle, A.T., Douglas, N.J. (1998) Comparison of nose and face mask CPAP therapy for sleep apnoea. *Thorax*, **53**, 290–2.

274 Massie, C.A., Hart, R.W., Peralez, K., Richards, G.N. (1999) Effects of humidification on nasal symptoms and compliance in sleep apnea patients using continuous positive airway pressure. *Chest*, **116**, 403–8.

275 Massie, C.A., Hart, R.W. (2000) Preliminary report on the comparison between automatic and manual positive airway pressure therapy in the home using the AutoSet T. *Sleep*, **23**, A264.

276 Teschler, H., Farhat, A.A., Exner, V., Konietzko, N., Berthon-Jones. M.

(1997) AutoSet nasal CPAP titration: constancy of pressure, compliance and effectiveness at 8 month follow-up. *Eur. Respir. J.*, **10**, 2073–8.

277 Meurice, J.C., Marc, I., Series, F. (1996) Efficacy of auto-CPAP in the treatment of obstructive sleep apnea/hypopnea syndrome. *Am. J. Respir. Crit. Care Med.*, **153**, 794–8.

278 Reeves-Hoche, M.K., Hudgel, D.W., Meck, R., Witteman, R., Ross, A., Zwillich, C.W. (1995) Continuous versus bilevel positive airway pressure for obstructive sleep apnea. *Am. J. Respir. Crit. Care Med.*, **151**, 443–9.

279 Stradling, J.R., Negus, T.W., Smith, D., Langford, B. (1998) Mandibular advancement devices for the control of snoring. *Eur. Respir. J.*, **11**, 447–50.

280 Ferguson, K.A., Ono, T., Lowe, A.A., Keenan, S.P., Fleetham, J.A. (1996) A randomized crossover study of an oral appliance vs nasal-continuous positive airway pressure in the treatment of mild-moderate obstructive sleep apnea. *Chest*, **109**, 1269–75.

281 Ferguson, K.A., Ono, T., Lowe, A.A., al-Majed, S., Love, L.L., Fleetham, J.A. (1997) A short-term controlled trial of an adjustable oral appliance for the treatment of mild to moderate obstructive sleep apnoea. *Thorax*, **52**, 362–8.

282 Schmidt-Nowara, W., Lowe, A., Wiegand, L., Cartwright, R., Perez-Guerra, F., Menn, S. (1995) Oral appliances for the treatment of snoring and obstructive sleep apnea: a review. *Sleep*, **18**, 501–10.

283 Bloch, K.E., Iseli, A., Zhang, J.N., Xie, X., Kaplan, V., Stoeckli, P.W. *et al.* (2000) A randomized, controlled crossover trial of two oral appliances for sleep apnea treatment. *Am. J. Respir. Crit. Care Med.*, **162**, 246–51.

284 Pantin, C.C., Hillman, D.R., Tennant, M. (1999) Dental side effects of an oral device to treat snoring and obstructive sleep apnea. *Sleep*, **22**, 237–40.

285 Engleman, H.M., McDonald, J.P., Graham, D., Lello, G.E., Kingshott, R.N., Coleman, E.L. *et al.* (2001) A randomized crossover trial of continuous positive airway pressure and mandibular repositioning slpint treatments for the sleep apnea/hypopnea syndrome. *Am. J. Respir. Crit. Care Med.*, **163**, A837.

286 Sher, A.E., Schechtman, K.B., Piccirillo, J.F. (1996) The efficacy of surgical modifications of the upper airway in adults with obstructive sleep apnea syndrome. *Sleep*, **19**, 156–77.

287 Pepin, J.L., Veale, D., Mayer, P., Bettega, G., Wuyam, B., Levy, P. (1996) Critical analysis of the results of surgery in the treatment of snoring, upper airway resistance syndrome (UARS), and obstructive sleep apnea (OSA). *Sleep*, **19**, S90–100.

288 Larsson, H., Carlsson-Nordlander, B., Svanborg, E. (1991) Long-time follow-up after UPPP for obstructive sleep apnea syndrome. Results of sleep apnea recordings and subjective evaluation 6 months and 2 years after surgery. *Acta Otolaryngol.*, **111**, 582–90.

289 Larsson, L.H., Carlsson-Nordlander, B., Svanborg, E. (1994) Four-year follow-up after uvulopalatopharyngoplasty in 50 unselected patients with obstructive sleep apnea syndrome. *Laryngoscope*, **104**, 1362–8.

290 Mortimore, I.L., Bradley, P.A., Murray, J.A., Douglas, N.J. (1996) Uvulopalatopharyngoplasty may compromise nasal CPAP therapy in sleep apnea syndrome. *Am. J. Respir. Crit. Care Med.*, **154**, 1759–62.

291 Walker, R.P., Grigg-Damberger, M.M., Gopalsami, C. (1997) Uvulopalatopharyngoplasty versus laser-assisted uvulopalatoplasty for the treatment of obstructive sleep apnea. *Laryngoscope*, **107**, 76–82.

292 Krespi, Y.P. (1998) The success of LAUP in select patients with sleep-related breathing disorders. *Arch. Otolaryngol. Head Neck Surg.*, **124**, 721.

293 Zohar, Y., Finkelstein, Y., Talmi, Y.P., Bar-Ilan, Y. (1991) Uvulopalatopharyngoplasty: evaluation of postoperative complications, sequelae, and results. *Laryngoscope*, **101**, 775–9.

294 Haavisto, L., Suonpaa, J. (1994) Complications of uvulopalatopharyngoplasty. *Clin. Otolaryngol.*, **19**, 243–7.

295 Haraldsson, P.O., Carenfelt, C., Lysdahl, M., Tingvall, C. (1995) Does uvulopalatopharyngoplasty inhibit automobile accidents? *Laryngoscope*, **105**, 657–61.

296 Woodson, B.T., Fujita, S. (1992) Clinical experience with lingualplasty as part of the treatment of severe obstructive sleep apnea. *Otolaryngol. Head Neck Surg.*, **107**, 40–8.

297 Fujita, S., Woodson, B.T., Clark, J.L., Wittig, R. (1991) Laser midline glossectomy as a treatment for obstructive sleep apnea. *Laryngoscope*, **101**, 805–9.

298 Riley, R.W., Powell, N.B., Guilleminault, C. (1994) Obstructive sleep apnea and the hyoid: a revised surgical procedure. *Otolaryngol. Head Neck Surg.*, **111**, 717–21.

299 Riley, R.W., Powell, N.B., Guilleminault, C. (1993) Obstructive sleep apnea syndrome: a review of 306 consecutively treated surgical patients. *Otolaryngol. Head Neck Surg.*, **108**, 117–25.

300 Series, F., St Pierre, S., Carrier, G. (1992) Effects of surgical correction of nasal obstruction in the treatment of obstructive sleep apnea. *Am. Rev. Respir. Dis.*, **146**, 1261–5.

301 Powell, N.B., Riley, R.W., Troell, R.J., Blumen, M.B., Guilleminault, C. (1997) Radiofrequency volumetric reduction of the tongue. A porcine pilot study for the treatment of obstructive sleep apnea syndrome. *Chest*, **111**, 1348–55.

302 Powell, N.B., Riley, R.W., Troell, R.J., Li, K., Blumen, M.B., Guilleminault, C. (1998) Radiofrequency volumetric tissue reduction of the palate in subjects with sleep-disordered breathing. *Chest*, **113**, 1163–74.

303 Boudewyns, A., Van De, H.P. (2000) Temperature-controlled radiofrequency tissue volume reduction of the soft palate (somnoplasty) in the treatment of habitual snoring: results of a European multicenter trial. *Acta Otolaryngol.*, **120**, 981–5.

304 Li, K.K., Powell, N.B., Riley, R.W., Troell, R.J., Guilleminault, C. (2000) Radiofrequency volumetric reduction of the palate: An extended follow- up study. *Otolaryngol. Head Neck Surg.*, **122**, 410–14.

305 Guilleminault, C., Quera-Salva, M.A., Powell, N.B., Riley, R.W. (1989) Maxillo-mandibular surgery for obstructive sleep apnoea. *Eur. Respir. J.*, **2**, 604–12.

306 Hochban, W., Brandenburg, U., Peter, J.H. (1994) Surgical treatment of obstructive sleep apnea by maxillomandibular advancement. *Sleep*, **17**, 624–9.

307 Conradt, R., Hochban, W., Heitmann, J., Brandenburg, U., Cassel, W., Penzel, T. *et al.* (1998) Sleep fragmentation and daytime vigilance in patients with OSA treated by surgical maxillomandibular advancement compared to CPAP therapy. *J. Sleep Res.*, 7, 217–23.

308 Conradt, R., Hochban, W., Brandenburg, U., Heitmann, J., Peter, J.H. (1997) Long-term follow-up after surgical treatment of obstructive sleep apnoea by maxillomandibular advancement. *Eur. Respir. J.*, **10**, 123–8.

309 Riley, R.W., Powell, N.B., Guilleminault, C. (1990) Maxillofacial surgery and nasal CPAP. A comparison of treatment for obstructive sleep apnea syndrome. *Chest*, **98**, 1421–5.

310 Eisele, D.W., Smith, P.L., Alam, D.S., Schwartz, A.R. (1997) Direct hypoglossal nerve stimulation in obstructive sleep apnea. *Arch. Otolaryngol. Head Neck Surg.*, **123**, 57–61.

311 Whyte, K.F., Gould, G.A., Airlie, M.A., Shapiro, C.M., Douglas, N.J. (1988) Role of protriptyline and acetazolamide in the sleep apnea/hypopnea syndrome. *Sleep*, **11**, 463–72.

312 Kingshott, R.N., Vennelle, M., Coleman, E.L., Engleman, H.M., Mackay, T.W., Douglas, N.J. (2001) Randomized, double-blind, placebo-controlled crossover trial of modafinil in the treatment of residual excessive daytime sleepiness in the sleep apnea/hypopnea syndrome. *Am. J. Respir. Crit. Care Med.*, **163**, 918–23.

313 Veasey, S.C., Chachkes, J., Fenik, P., Hendricks, J.C. (2001) The effects of ondansetron on sleep-disordered breathing in the English bulldog. *Sleep*, **24**, 155–60.

314 Kryger, M.H., Roos, L., Delaive, K., Walld, R., Horrocks, J. (1996)

Utilization of health care services in patients with severe obstructive sleep apnea. *Sleep*, **19**, S111–16.

315 Kapur, V., Blough, D.K., Sandblom, R.E., Hert, R., de Maine, J.B., Sullivan, S.D. *et al.* (1999) The medical cost of undiagnosed sleep apnea. *Sleep*, **22**, 749–55.

316 Ronald, J., Delaive, K., Roos, L., Manfreda, J., Bahammam, A., Kryger, M.H. (1999) Health care utilization in the 10 years prior to diagnosis in obstructive sleep apnea syndrome patients. *Sleep*, **22**, 225–9.

317 Peker, Y., Hedner, J., Johansson, A., Bende, M. (1997) Reduced hospitalization with cardiovascular and pulmonary disease in obstructive sleep apnea patients on nasal CPAP treatment. *Sleep*, **20**, 645–53.

318 Bahammam, A., Delaive, K., Ronald, J., Manfreda, J., Roos, L,. Kryger, M.H. (1999) Health care utilization in males with obstructive sleep apnea syndrome two years after diagnosis and treatment. *Sleep*, **22**, 740–7.

319 Tousignant, P., Cosio, M.G., Levy, R.D., Groome, P.A. (1994) Quality adjusted life years added by treatment of obstructive sleep apnea. *Sleep*, **17**, 52–60.

320 Chilcott, J., Clayton, E., Chada, N., Hanning, C.D., Kinnear, W., Waterhouse, J.C. (2000) *Nasal Continuous Positive Airways Pressure in the Management of Sleep Apnoea*. Leicester: Trent Institute for Health Services Research.

Narcolepsy

Introduction

Narcolepsy is an uncommon but important disorder characterized by marked daytime sleepiness sometimes in conjunction with cataplexy, the loss of postural muscle tone in response to emotional stimuli. Narcolepsy is under-diagnosed and many sufferers may never realize the cause of their disabling symptoms nor receive appropriate advice or therapy. One of the major challenges facing sleep medicine is to rectify this situation.

History

The term 'narcolepsy' was coined in 1880 by the French neuropsychiatrist Gelineau who detailed two cases, one a 36-year-old man described as having numerous sleep attacks and falling over when dealt a good hand at cards.[1] There was considerable scepticism from many physicians about the presence of this condition, with some believing it was merely a manifestation of hysteria. However, gradually increasing numbers of clear-cut cases were reported until it became clear by 1926 that narcolepsy was a genuine medical condition.[2]

Aetiology

Narcolepsy results from dysfunction within the central nervous system but the precise deficit has not yet been found, although major advances are being made and a functional defect of hypocretin is almost certainly the key component.

Most cases of narcolepsy are idiopathic but there have been a few case reports of narcolepsy developing in association with brain lesions, including tumours, trauma, multiple sclerosis and pontine gliosis.[3,4] A review of 16 cases of narcolepsy associated with known brain pathology concluded that brainstem lesions were the likely common factor,[5] although hypothalamic and pituitary lesions have also been associated.[3] However, in the far more common form of idiopathic narcolepsy, extensive searching has failed to identify any evidence of consistent focal neuropathological lesions.

FAMILIAL NARCOLEPSY IN HUMANS

There is a familial element to narcolepsy, but it is not as strong as many believed. Although approximately six to seven per cent of first-degree relatives of patients with narcolepsy give a story of daytime sleepiness, only 15/334 relatives of patients with narcolepsy with cataplexy were proven to have narcolepsy with cataplexy, giving a frequency of narcolepsy of 0.9 per cent in the first-degree relatives of cases of definite narcolepsy.[6] This is, nevertheless, significantly higher than the frequency of narcolepsy in the community – see below – indicating an uncommon but genuine familial tendency for the condition.

Several twin studies have been performed, but cast little light on the mechanism of inheritance of the condition. Less than a third of the monozygotic twin pairs reported are concordant for narcolepsy with cataplexy.[7] However, it is difficult to draw firm conclusions from this, as not all studies show the same degree of diagnostic rigour and few report long-term follow-up of unaffected twins to demonstrate whether narcolepsy develops later in one twin. There is a clear need for further studies. As human narcolepsy is rarely familial and twin studies show a high rate of discordance, environmental factors are important in human narcolepsy.[7]

EVIDENCE FROM ANIMAL STUDIES OF GENE DEFECTS

Some strains of Doberman Pinscher dogs have familial narcolepsy with sleepiness and cataplexy. This is transmitted as an autosomal recessive and the gene defect has been identified as a deletion in the transcript of the hypocretin type 2 receptor, Hcrtr2.[8] Hcrt gene knock-out mice exhibit episodes of behavioural arrest which may represent cataplexy.[9] Hypocretins – also called orexins – are expressed by neurones in the lateral hypothalamus which project into the brainstem and forebrain. The lateral hypothalamic region in which the Hcrt neurones are found is believed to be the 'appetite control centre'. Hcrt-producing cells express leptin receptor immunoreactivity and genetically obese mice have downregulated Hcrt gene expression. Micro-injection of Hcrt induces feeding and increases basal metabolic rate.[10]

HYPOCRETINS IN HUMAN NARCOLEPSY

Unlike dogs, most humans with narcolepsy do not have abnormalities in the genes controlling hypocretin 2 receptor production.[11] However, hypocretin levels were undetectable in the cerebrospinal fluid (CSF) of seven of nine patients with narcolepsy.[12] A study of narcoleptic brains has found that hypocretin producing neurones were reduced by approximately 90 per cent in narcoleptic hypothalami.[13] Thus decreased hypocretin production seems to be a major factor in human narcolepsy.

HLA TYPE

Narcolepsy is reported to be the medical condition most closely linked to human leucocyte antigen (HLA) type. Over 85 per cent of Caucasians and Japanese narcoleptic individuals are HLA DR2 DQw1 positive.[14,15] However, in Afro-Americans DR2 occurs in only 75 per cent of narcoleptic patients, whereas the association with DQw1 is as strong as in Caucasians.[16]

These observations have been refined with genomic mapping of the HLA regions on chromosome 6. Studies of the DQw1 region show that the DQB1*0602 allele is closely linked with narcolepsy across ethnic groups and is positive in 84–95 per cent of narcoleptic subjects with clear cataplexy.[14,17] The linkage is weaker in patients without cataplexy who were labelled as narcoleptics, in whom only 41 per cent were DQB1*0602.[17] DQB1*0602 is present in approximately 22 per cent of the normal Caucasian and 40 per cent of the normal Black population[17] and so is of little diagnostic specificity. Interestingly, DQB1*0602 may be associated with short sleep latency in normal subjects,[18] although this awaits independent confirmation. Overall, the best association with narcolepsy across ethnic groups appears to be with DQB1*0602 and DQA1*0102.[19,20]

There is no evidence as yet of any difference in DNA sequence in the DQB1*0602, DQA1*0102 region within the HLA region of chromosome 6 between narcoleptic and normal subjects.[16,19,21] Although the entire gene in the HLA DQ regions has been sequenced, no candidate gene other than the DQA1*0102 and DQB1*0602 genes has been found.[19]

The reason why narcolepsy is so closely linked to HLA type is unknown. The genes encoding for HLA DR are located within the major histocompatability complex (MHC) Class II region. These HLA Class II molecules are transmembrane glycoprotein heterodimers which each have an alpha and beta chain – DRA and DRB for DR; DQA1 and DQB1 for DQ – and are usually expressed on the surface of B-cells and macrophages, where they bind antigens and present them to T-cells. The gene system involved in the association of HLA DQB1*0602 with narcolepsy thus probably plays a role in the immune response and so it has been suggested that narcolepsy may be an autoimmune disorder, like most other diseases with an HLA association.[22] However, extensive examination of the blood, CSF and brain tissue of patients with narcolepsy have failed to identify any evidence of an autoimmune process,[23–25] so the significance of this association remains unknown.

MECHANISM OF NARCOLEPSY IN HUMANS – CONCLUSIONS

The association of narcolepsy with HLA types has led to the suggestion that it is an auto-immune disease which results in destruction of hypocretin-producing cells, analogous to insulin-dependent diabetes, but this is unproven.[20,26] However, there are unpublished reports that hypocretin levels may be normal in some families with narcolepsy, and these combined with a single case report[11] suggest that some families or cases may, like the dobermans, have a receptor defect. Thus it seems likely that narcolepsy may result from multiple different abnormalities, in either the hypocretin production or hypocretin receptor systems producing the same clinical syndrome. It is likely that the vast majority are acquired, with destruction of hypocretin production in HLA predisposed individuals following an unknown trigger, but a few cases are due to inherited or spontaneous defects in hypocretin receptors or possibly hypocretin production.

Epidemiology

There are wide differences in the reported frequencies of narcolepsy between different studies with reported prevalences per 10,000 population ranging from 0.02[27] to 59.[28] There are several possible reasons for these differences, including strictness of diagnosis, study size, diligence of case ascertainment and ethnicity. As usual the truth lies probably somewhere between the extreme figures with estimates of cases per 10,000 population among Caucasians of two,[29] three,[30] four[31] and five.[32] Thus, a working figure of four narcoleptic subjects per 10,000 Caucasian population is reasonable, but the confidence limits of the estimates from all these studies are wide with many ranging at least from 0 to 12 cases per 10,000.

The influence of race on the prevalence of narcolepsy is not clear. Estimates in Black Americans approximate those in Caucasians. Studies in Japanese have suggested a high prevalence ranging from 16 to 59 cases per 10,000.[28] A study from Israel has suggested a very low prevalence of 0.02 per 10,000 population,[27] one-thousandth of that reported from Japan. It seems unlikely that the racial differences are truly that large, and methodological and diagnostic differences could be major factors. There is thus a need for larger studies with more precise diagnostic categorization.

AGE OF ONSET

Increasingly, it is being recognized that the clinical features of narcolepsy begin in childhood or adolescence in many, perhaps most, patients.[33] However, because the delay between symptom onset and diagnosis is usually several years, most are not diagnosed until early adulthood. Onset over the age of 50 is unusual.

SEX RATIO

There is no striking sex difference in prevalence, although some have said that males are affected slightly more often than females.

Clinical features

Sleepiness and cataplexy are the two most characteristic symptoms of narcolepsy. Cataplexy is a manifestation of REM phenomena intruding into wakefulness, as are also sleep paralysis and hallucinations at sleep onset.

SLEEPINESS

The sleepiness is most marked in the usual soporific situations, such as after meals, in the afternoon or evening, in warm surroundings and monotonous situations. However, a typical feature of narcolepsy is the ability to fall asleep in unusual as well as usual circumstances, such as standing, walking, cycling, skiing and during intercourse. Normally, sleep episodes come on gradually with warning, however sometimes they can be sudden and without warning. Sleep attacks can often be delayed to some extent voluntarily, although this may be at the expense of extreme irritability. Many sleep attacks last 10–30 minutes but there is a wide range from a few seconds to several hours. Most patients report one to six naps per day, but there may also be many more brief and unnoticed microsleeps. Any factor which can make normal subjects more sleepy – including sleep deprivation, hypnotic or sedative drugs and alcohol – will tend to worsen the hypersomnolence.

Naps may or may not be refreshing, although classical teaching was that the naps were refreshing. As well as being afflicted by the sleep episodes many patients find they are abnormally drowsy, spending much of the day in a sub-alert state that influences their work performance and memory.

CATAPLEXY

Cataplexy is a sudden decrease or loss of voluntary muscle tone usually precipitated by emotion, particularly laughter, surprise or anger. Typically, the jaw drops, the head nods, the arms drop to the side and the knees sag. The presence of facial twitching during attacks is a useful pointer in favour of cataplexy.[34] Attacks may be localized or generalized and in some patients the typical attack may be limited to head nodding. Some attacks appear to involve all voluntary muscle groups and result in absolute powerlessness and complete collapse, although injury is rare. Cataplexy is almost always bilateral, but approximately one per cent of cases may be unilateral.[35] Cataplectic episodes usually last only a few seconds but can last up to 10 minutes. Usually, awareness continues normally throughout attacks. Cataplectic attacks may be mistaken for epilepsy.[36]

Laughter is the most common cause of cataplexy, but fear, intense concentration, coughing and sneezing may also initiate attacks. Physical effort may also be a trigger, and this combined with the anticipation of imminent achievement often makes sport a major problem for cataplectic patients – for example the professional soccer player who fell over from cataplexy every time he got excited because he thought he was going to score a goal!

HYPNAGOGIC HALLUCINATIONS

Such hallucinations at sleep onset constitute one part of the classical narcoleptic tetrad of sleepiness, cataplexy, hypnagogic hallucinations and sleep paralysis. The hallucinations take place in the twilight zone between wakefulness and sleep and may occur when sleep is being fought. They are vivid dream episodes that may take any visual form found in dreams, but there is usually some sort of awareness of the surroundings. Sometimes there may be auditory hallucinations, and these may falsely give rise to concern about the presence of schizophrenia. These hallucinations are assumed to reflect the propensity of narcoleptic subjects to go rapidly into REM sleep.

However, whether hypnagogic hallucinations are truly a feature of narcolepsy has been questioned, as they occur frequently in other sleep disorders.[37] Certainly, occasional hallucinations are not diagnostically useful, but hypnagogic hallucinations occurring regularly several times per week are suggestive of narcolepsy. Sometimes the hallucinations may happen on wakening when they are termed 'hypnopompic'.

SLEEP PARALYSIS

Wakening unable to move is a frightening experience, particularly the first time it occurs. The ability to move returns after a variable period, often seconds but sometimes a few minutes. Sleep paralysis can occur in normal subjects, particularly in young adults and those with irregular sleep times. Occasionally, sleep paralysis may run in families in the absence of other evidence of any illness. The absence of sleep paralysis does not exclude the diagnosis of narcolepsy, and sleep paralysis also occurs in a variety of other sleep disorders.[37]

AUTOMATIC BEHAVIOUR

Episodes of amnesia associated with semi-purposeful behaviour may happen in up to 40 per cent of narcoleptics. The cause is unknown but may be due to impaired vigilance due to sleepiness, microsleeps or REM sleep intrusion into wakefulness. These episodes may range from sudden bursts of meaningless, disconnected speech, writing rubbish in the middle of an otherwise well-composed script, ignoring traffic signals or driving on the wrong side of the road. The patient usually has little or no memory for the attacks. Such episodes are not pathognomonic of narcolepsy and may occur in any disorder causing severe chronic sleepiness. Ataxia accompanied by automatic behaviour occurs in around 10 per cent of narcoleptic subjects and is termed 'sleep drunkenness'.

INSOMNIA

Insomnia is a problem for many patients with narcolepsy. Around three-quarters of narcoleptic subjects report frequent awakenings, light sleep or unsatisfying sleep.[38] Indeed, the difficulty maintaining sleep may be so severe that patients may originally be diagnosed as having daytime sleepiness resulting from their insomnia, and some are initially treated with hypnotics.

PARASOMNIAS

Narcoleptics have an increased frequency of sleep talking and sleep walking. These may be significant problems for some patients.

EFFECTS ON DAYTIME FUNCTION

Narcolepsy has marked effects on daytime performance and is associated with a high rate of work-related difficulties. Broughton *et al.*[39] found that among 148 working narcoleptic subjects, work problems related to sleep attacks were reported by 95 per cent. Other difficulties were inability to concentrate (43 per cent), memory problems (31 per cent) and interpersonal problems (24 per cent). A third reported other people did not understand or were intolerant of their problems, often viewing them as lazy. Half were fearful of job loss and a similar number felt they had decreased earnings or been passed over for promotion because of their narcolepsy.

There are limited objective data on daytime performance in narcoleptics. Mean reaction time was almost twice as long in a group of narcoleptic compared with matched control subjects[40] and the narcoleptics had four times as many very delayed responses as the control subjects, a feature which might be vital in driving performance. When narcoleptics were allowed to nap through the day their performance improved significantly, but was still closer to that of non-napping narcoleptics than to controls.

Problems in the home are also common. Three-quarters of narcoleptic subjects reported marital and family problems, and 40 per cent said their narcolepsy created tension in the family.[41] Sexual dysfunction is also blamed on narcolepsy. Seventeen per cent of both sexes reported a decrease in sex drive since onset of their narcolepsy and impotence was reported by 15 per cent compared to four per cent of control subjects.[39] In some impotence may result from therapy, for example with tricyclics.

In children with narcolepsy, schooling can pose major challenges. Half of 360 narcoleptic subjects believed that their symptoms were the reason for poor grades at school.[39] A third blamed their narcolepsy for poor relationships with their teachers. Social isolation is a major risk which needs to be handled with care.

Overall quality of life is markedly impaired in narcoleptics.[39,42,43] Even when taking treatment, quality of life remains significantly impaired for most.

DRIVING

Patients with narcolepsy are at increased risk of automobile accidents. Broughton and colleagues[39] found that 66 per cent of narcoleptics reported falling asleep at the wheel as opposed to six per cent of control subjects. Accidents as a result of sleepiness were reported by 37 per cent of narcoleptics compared with five per cent of controls. Cataplexy when driving occurred in 29 per cent of narcoleptics.

Performance on a 'driving simulator' computerized vigilance task in which subjects have to avoid objects during a boring 30-minute 'drive' is impaired in patients with narcolepsy.[44] The narcoleptics hit more objects than age- and sex-matched control subjects. In addition, the narcoleptic individuals whose performance was poor on this 'SteerClear' test had a significantly higher automobile accident rate than those whose SteerClear performance was normal. Studies on a more sophisticated driving simulator also confirmed that narcoleptics drive much worse than control subjects[45] (Figure 3.1). Interestingly, there was no close correlation between the performance on SteerClear or the driving simulator and the patient's multiple sleep latency test (MSLT) result.

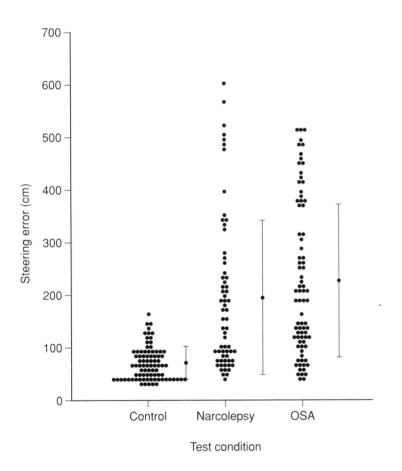

Figure 3.1
Steering error on a driving simulator in normal controls is less than in narcoleptics or obstructive sleep apnoea/hypopnoea syndrome (OSA) patients. (Adapted from George,[45] with permission.)

Course and prognosis

The symptoms of narcolepsy often come on gradually. In about 80 per cent of patients sleepiness is the first symptom to develop, with cataplexy the first in approximately 10 per cent of patients.[29] The other features may come on several years after the start of the initial symptom.

Once symptoms have started, they usually persist for the rest of the patient's life. Narcolepsy only rarely ceases with age, but cataplexy has been reported to stop spontaneously in up to 20 per cent of cases. In one study, approximately 90 per cent of patients had a relatively stable course to their disease with 10 per cent having intermittent remissions and relapses.[29] Variations in severity may depend on mood, sleep deprivation, drug therapy and alcohol, although climate has also been blamed.

Investigation

There is no gold standard test for narcolepsy. Diagnostic methods and their limitations are discussed in Chapter 5. History is very important in making the diagnosis, but alone is not sufficient to give individuals a life-long label and give them life-long therapy. HLA testing is not of sufficient diagnostic specificity or sensitivity to be clinically helpful.

Overnight sleep testing is needed in patients in whom the story suggests other possible diagnoses, and this usually means in snorers. In North America, polysomnography is standard in patients with possible narcolepsy, usually followed by an MSLT. Diagnostic criteria thereafter may vary.[46,47]

In our centre, those with cataplexy plus sleepiness are studied principally by an MSLT. In this group a mean sleep latency of less than eight minutes with at least one sleep onset REM sleep (SOREMs) is regarded as diagnostic.

In patients who have possible narcolepsy without cataplexy, the diagnostic criteria for narcolepsy should be more strict. Thus we perform polysomnography on these patients – to exclude OSAHS and periodic limb movement disorder (PLMD) – and then an MSLT. Those with a normal polysomnography and a mean sleep latency of less than eight minutes with two SOREMs – and no other reasons for SOREMs (*see* page 143) – may be diagnosed as having narcolepsy without cataplexy.

Treatment

The self-evident aim is to allow narcoleptic patients to lead as normal a life as possible. Physicians caring for narcoleptics must ensure that adequate attention is paid to the importance of non-pharmacological approaches as well as to drug therapy. There is an understandable desire among some physicians and patients to seek a simple pharmacological solution to all aspects of the condition, but medication alone is insufficient. Advice is required on lifestyle alterations and measures to minimize symptoms. In addition, time must be spent educating newly diagnosed patients about the medico-legal and familial aspects of the condition. Provision of web-based information –

PEANUTS

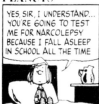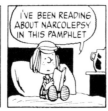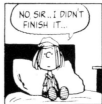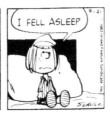

Figure 3.2
Charlie Brown's view of narcolepsy leaflets. (*International Herald Tribune*, 1983, with permission.)

such as the British Sleep Foundation (www.britishsleepfoundation.org.uk), National Sleep Foundation (www.sleepfoundation.org) or Sleep Home Pages (www.sleephomepages.org) – and easy to read educational leaflets (Figure 3.2) are helpful.

NON-PHARMACOLOGICAL APPROACHES

Nocturnal sleep
Patients should be encouraged to maintain a normal nocturnal sleep duration and avoid activities which will result in sleep deprivation. Sleep restriction increases narcoleptic symptoms.[48] Narcoleptic patients reporting impaired night-time sleep describe increased need for daytime naps.[49] Extending the nocturnal sleep duration of narcoleptics has been reported to decrease their daytime symptoms.[33]

Daytime naps
Planned naps during the day are a standard component of therapy for narcolepsy, indeed, many patients institute regular naps even before the diagnosis is made. Naps help both subjective and objective sleepiness with improvements of approximately 33–100 per cent in the maintenance of wakefulness test (MWT) following protocols of two or three planned 15-minute naps a day.[50] Roehrs *et al.*[51] found that 15-minute naps were as good as 30-minute naps in improving sleep latency on the MSLT. Naps improve not only sleepiness but also daytime performance, including reaction time.[40,52]

Diet
Alcohol avoidance or minimization is of benefit to narcoleptics. Although alcohol suppresses REM sleep, this is followed by a rebound increase in REM sleep tendency which may worsen cataplexy.

Caffeine ingestion in tea, coffee and colas is commonly used by sufferers to aid alertness. Six cups of strong coffee are said to have similar stimulant effects to 5 mg of dexamphetamine.[53]

Occupation

By the time the diagnosis is made it is often unrealistic to make major changes to the occupation of the patient. However, those diagnosed in their teens or early adult life should be informed that monotonous sedentary jobs are often difficult for narcoleptic individuals to perform. They should also be steered away from occupations involving driving or dangerous machinery. Most subjects with milder narcolepsy can manage occupations involving continuous activity, especially if in a stimulating environment.

PHARMACOLOGICAL AGENTS

For sleepiness

A range of stimulant drugs is used in patients with narcolepsy to reduce their daytime sleepiness. Patients vary considerably in their responses to different agents and in their development of side-effects. As a result there is no single stimulant of choice, rather there are options, several of which may need to be tried before adequate clinical control is achieved without intolerable side-effects.

The mechanism of action of these drugs varies. However, many work by increasing noradrenaline or dopamine levels in the synaptic cleft.[54] There is no consensus about the order in which stimulants should be tried. Most would agree that amphetamines are not the agents of first choice; effective as they can be, their side-effect profile and potential for abuse makes them suitable for use only if there has been no satisfactory response to two or more other agents.

Non-amphetamines

Modafinil

Modafinil is a relatively new drug which has been used in France since the early 1980s but has only recently become more widely available. Its precise mode of action is unclear, but does not appear to be through either dopaminergic or noradrenergic mechanisms.[55,56] Modafinil is the wakefulness-promoting drug which has the greatest evidence of efficacy from well-conducted randomized controlled trials. These studies carried out in Europe,[57] Canada[58] and the USA[59,60] have all shown reduction in symptoms and in both subjective and objective sleepiness compared to placebo. Although there were highly statistically significant improvements with modafinil over placebo, there is a total lack of any data comparing efficacy with other stimulants. These data are being generated now and should clarify the precise role of modafinil. However, because of proven efficacy, relatively few side-effects and low abuse potential[59,60] modafinil is one of the agents of first choice at present. Modafinil is safe in overdose, one patient who took 45 100 mg tablets had no medical sequelae except for sleeplessness (Kreiger J, personal communication). Modafinil has no effect on cataplexy.

Mazindol

Mazindol is an imadazoline derivative which has been shown to reduce sleepiness in narcoleptic subjects.[61] In the usual daily dosages of 2–6 mg cardiovascular side-effects are unusual. Tolerance to mazindol may occur but is relatively unusual and abuse is rare. Mazindol is more often used in Europe than in North America.

Selegiline

This monoamine oxidase type B inhibitor can be effective against both the sleepiness and cataplectic features. A dose of 40 mg/day produced a 36 per cent reduction in the number of daytime sleep episodes and a 89 per cent fall in cataplectic attacks in one study.[62]

Gamma hydroxybutyrate

This naturally occurring metabolite is a relatively newly tried agent which has both weak stimulant and weak hypnotic effects when taken at night.[63] In this controlled trial it had no significant anti-cataplectic effect, but further studies are under way.

Amphetamines

Dexamphetamine

Dexamphetamine is a powerful central nervous system stimulant which will increase vigilance, decrease sleep and elevate mood and can be very effective in narcolepsy.[64] Unfortunately, side-effects are limiting in many patients, in particular anxiety, headache, anorexia, nausea and sweating. Tolerance develops in many patients and some benefit from breaks in therapy – 'drug holidays'. As amphetamines are both abused and addictive, care has to be taken that they do not fall into the wrong hands through either patients with narcolepsy or patients feigning narcolepsy.

Methylphenidate

Methylphenidate is a piperadine derivative related to amphetamine but with fewer side-effects and more rapid onset of action. Indeed some, particularly in North America, consider methylphenidate to be the stimulant of choice in patients with narcolepsy.[65] The studies on methylphenidate are largely not randomized or controlled, but the data suggest similar efficacy to amphetamine.[64] Methylphenidate has been reported to improve sleepiness in over 90 per cent of patients and help cataplexy in over 80 per cent. Improvement was dose-related and greatest in those taking more than 60 mg per day. The most common side-effects were dry mouth, headache, abdominal discomfort, sweating and difficulties with micturition.

Pemoline

Pemoline is pharmacologically similar to amphetamine, however, it is a less potent stimulant than either amphetamine or methylphenidate.[64] Pemoline is usually used in dosages of 37.5 mg to up to 200 mg per day. Two-thirds of patients treated with pemoline alone and followed for eight years reported at least moderate improvements in their sleepiness. Stomach discomfort, anorexia, mouth dryness and headaches were the major side-effects reported. Liver function abnormalities developing on treatment have lead to a decrease in pemoline usage and restrictions on its availability in some countries, including the UK and the USA. Pemoline should now be used with extreme caution or not at all, and not as a first-line drug.

Relative potencies of stimulants

There are few data comparing drugs (Table 3.1). Mitler and colleagues[66] tried to compare some agent efficacies from published data (Figure 3.3).

Drug holidays

Long-term use of high doses of stimulants, particularly of amphetamines, can give rise to habituation and rising dosage needs. Some patients can usefully reset their dosage requirements by taking a one- or two-week drug holiday.

REM sleep intrusion phenomena

If the REM intrusion phenomena are mild and the patient is being started on a stimulant which has anti-cataplexy effects, it is prudent to see whether

Table 3.1
Stimulant drugs for narcolepsy

Agent	Daily dose (mg)	Tablet size (mg)	Half-life (hours)	Potency
Modafinil	200–400	100	6	+
Mazindol	2–8	2	2	+
Methylphenidate	10–60	10	2	+ +
Dexamphetamine	5–60	5	12	+ + +
Other drugs				
Selegiline	10–40 mg/day			
Gammahydroxybutyrate	3–9 mg/day at bedtime			

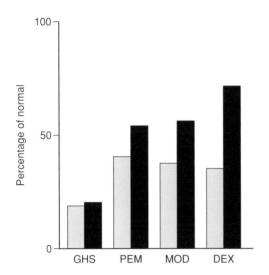

Relative eddicacy of drugs for treating narcolepsy

Percentage of normal

Figure 3.3
Comparative efficacy of stimulents in narcolepsy. Grey areas represent baseline sleepiness where 100 per cent represents normal alertness; dark areas represent sleepiness on treatment. GHB = gammahydroxybutyrate; PEM = pemoline; MOD = modafinil; DEX = dexamphetamine. (Adapted from Mitler,[66] with permission.)

the stimulant produces adequate control on its own before embarking on other more specific treatment. Cataplexy, sleep-related hallucinations and sleep paralysis are all helped by agents which suppress REM sleep. Most commonly these are antidepressants, tricyclics, quadricyclics or selective serotinegic reuptake inhibitors (SSRIs). SSRIs are the current treatment of choice. The mechanism of action of these drugs is believed to be by blocking noradrenaline reuptake, thus increasing its concentration in the synaptic cleft.

Many patients will need to be tried on more than one REM sleep inhibitor to obtain optimal benefit/side-effect ratio. It is essential that the patients are fully educated about the rationale for use of these drugs as insufficient explanation may result in the belief that they are being used to treat their depression and poor compliance can result.

SSRIs
- Fluoxetine: 20–60 mg daily taken in the morning is my routine initial treatment for cataplexy.
- Viloxazine: 50–200 mg daily taken in two divided doses.
- Venlafaxine: 150–300 mg in the morning.

Others
- Clomipramine: 25–200 mg daily.
- Protriptyline: 2.5–20 mg daily.

Driving regulations

The rules governing driving for people with narcolepsy vary between countries. In the UK, the onus is on drivers to report their sleepiness when driving and their diagnosis of narcolepsy to the licensing authorities. A sleep specialist or neurologist is then usually asked to provide a medical report on the patient's fitness to drive. Narcoleptics who are well-controlled are often allowed to drive cars but are generally not allowed to drive trucks or buses.

Unfortunately, in most countries there is no specific advice about the objective criteria to be met before a patient may drive. For example, no attempt has been made to allow patients to drive if they reach specific levels of alertness on the MSLT or MWT or specific performances on a driving simulator test. In some states in the USA and in many other countries, a history of adequate narcoleptic control is the major determinant of whether driving is allowed to resume. However, this approach is potentially flawed with risk of non-disclosure of sleepiness or accidents. Further, the assumption is made that once patients are established on therapy they will unfailingly continue to take it, is naïve in the extreme if the experience of other chronic conditions is to taken into account.[67]

The position of confidentiality between the doctor and the driving authorities differs between countries. A recent recommendation from the General Medical Council[68] in the UK has indicated that doctors who believe their patients are driving against medical advice should notify the medical advisors to the Driving and Vehicle Licensing Authority. Although the rationale for this is understandable, there is a risk that patients with severe narcolepsy who need to drive for their living may be deterred from seeking medical help if they realize that information about their illness may be passed on without their permission. There is thus a risk that this could result in more – rather than fewer – sleepy drivers on the roads.

References

1 Gellineau, J.B. (1880) De la narcolepsie. *Gaz Hop (Paris)*, 53, 626–37.
2 Adie, W.J. (1926) Idiopathic narcolepsy: a disease *sui generis*: with remarks on the mechanisms of sleep. *Brain*, 49, 257–306.
3 Aldrich, M.S., Naylor, M.W. (1989) Narcolepsy associated with lesions of the diencephalon. *Neurology*, **39**, 1505–8.
4 Stahl, S.M., Layzer, R.B., Aminoff, M.J., Townsend, J.J., Feldon, S. (1980) Continuous cataplexy in a patient with a midbrain tumor: the limp man syndrome. *Neurology*, **30**, 1115–18.

5   Clavelou, P., Tournilhac, M., Vidal, C., Georget, A.M., Picard, L., Merienne, L. (1995) Narcolepsy associated with arteriovenous malformation of the diencephalon. *Sleep*, **18**, 202–5.

6   Guilleminault, C., Mignot, E., Grumet, F.C. (1989) Familial patterns of narcolepsy. *Lancet*, **2**, 1376–9.

7   Mignot, E. (1998) Genetic and familial aspects of narcolepsy. *Neurology*, **50**, S16–22.

8   Lin, L., Faraco, J., Li, R., Kadotani, H., Rogers, W., Lin, X. *et al.* (1999) The sleep disorder canine narcolepsy is caused by a mutation in the hypocretin (orexin) receptor 2 gene. *Cell*, **98**, 365–76.

9   Chemelli, R.M., Willie, J.T., Sinton, C.M., Elmquist, J.K., Scammell, T., Lee, C. *et al.* (1999) Narcolepsy in orexin knockout mice: molecular genetics of sleep regulation. *Cell*, **98**, 437–51.

10 Sweet, D.C., Levine, A.S., Billington, C.J., Kotz, C.M. (1999) Feeding response to central orexins. *Brain Res.*, **821**, 535–8.

11 Peyron, C., Faraco, J., Rogers, W., Ripley, B., Overeem, S., Charnay, Y. *et al.* (2000) A mutation in a case of early onset narcolepsy and a generalized absence of hypocretin peptides in human narcoleptic brains. *Nat. Med.*, **6**, 991–7.

12 Nishino, S., Ripley, B., Overeem, S., Lammers, G.J., Mignot, E. (2000) Hypocretin (orexin) deficiency in human narcolepsy. *Lancet*, **355**, 39–40.

13 Thannickal, T.C., Moore, R.Y., Neinhuis, R., Ramanathan, L., Gulyani, S., Aldrich, M. *et al.* (2000) Reduced number of hypocretin neurons in human narcolepsy. *Neuron.*, **27**, 469–74.

14 Rogers, A.E., Meehan, J., Guilleminault, C., Grumet, F.C., Mignot, E. (1997) HLA DR15 (DR2) and DQB1*0602 typing studies in 188 narcoleptic patients with cataplexy. *Neurology*, **48**, 1550–6.

15 Langdon, N., Welsh, K.I., van Dam, M., Vaughan, R.W., Parkes, D. (1984) Genetic markers in narcolepsy. *Lancet*, **2**, 1178–80.

16 Mignot, E., Lin, X., Arrigoni, J., Macaubas, C., Olive, F., Hallmayer, J. *et al.* (1994) DQB1*0602 and DQA1*0102 (DQ1) are better markers than DR2 for narcolepsy in Caucasian and black Americans. *Sleep*, **17**, S607.

17 Mignot, E., Hayduk, R., Black, J., Grumet, F.C., Guilleminault, C. (1997) HLA DQB1*0602 is associated with cataplexy in 509 narcoleptic patients. *Sleep*, **20**, 1012–20.

18 Mignot, E., Young, T., Lin, L., Finn, L., Palta, M. (1998) Reduction of REM sleep latency associated with HLA-DQB1*0602 in normal adults [letter]. *Lancet*, **351**, 727.

19 Mignot, E., Kimura, A., Lattermann, A., Lin, X., Yasunaga, S., Mueller-Eckhardt, G. *et al.* (1997) Extensive HLA class II studies in 58 non-DRB1*15 (DR2) narcoleptic patients with cataplexy. *Tissue Antigens*, **49**, 329–41.

20   Mignot, E., Lin, L., Rogers, W., Honda, Y., Qiu, X., Lin, X. *et al.* (2001) Complex HLA-DR and -DQ interactions confer risk of narcolepsy–cataplexy in three ethnic groups. *Am. J. Hum. Genet.*, **68**, 686–99.

21   Uryu, N., Maeda, M., Nagata, Y., Matsuki, K., Juji, T., Honda, Y. *et al.* (1989) No difference in the nucleotide sequence of the DQ beta beta 1 domain between narcoleptic and healthy individuals with DR2,Dw2. *Hum. Immunol.*, **24**, 175–81.

22   Parkes, J.D., Langdon, N., Lock, C. (1986) Narcolepsy and immunity [editorial]. *BMJ*, **292**, 359–60.

23   Erlich, S.S., Itabashi, H.H. (1986) Narcolepsy: a neuropathologic study. *Sleep*, **9**, 126–32.

24   Fredrikson, S., Carlander, B., Billiard, M., Link, H. (1990) CSF immune variables in patients with narcolepsy. *Acta Neurol. Scand.*, **81**, 253–4.

25   Carlander, B., Eliaou, J.F., Billiard, M. (1993) Autoimmune hypothesis in narcolepsy. *Neurophysiol. Clin.*, **23**, 15–22.

26   Mignot, E. (2000) Perspectives in narcolepsy and hypocretin (orexin) research. *Sleep Medicine*, **1**, 87–90.

27   Wilner, A., Steinman, L., Lavie, P., Peled, R., Friedmann, A., Brautbar, C. (1988) Narcolepsy–cataplexy in Israeli Jews is associated exclusively with the HLA DR2 haplotype. A study at the serological and genomic level. *Hum. Immunol.*, **21**, 15–22.

28   Tashiro, T., Kanbayashi, T., Iijima, S., Hishikawa, Y. (1992) An epidemiological study on prevalence of narcolepsy in Japanese. *J. Sleep Res.*, **1**, 228 (abstract).

29   Roth, B. (1980) *Narcolepsy and Hypersomnia.* Basel: Karger.

30   Hublin, C., Partinen, M., Kaprio, J., Koskenvuo, M., Guilleminault, C. (1994) Epidemiology of narcolepsy. *Sleep*, 17, S7–12.

31   Franceschi, M., Zamproni, P., Crippa, D., Smirne, S. (1982) Excessive daytime sleepiness: a 1-year study in an unselected inpatient population. *Sleep*, **5**, 239–47.

32   Dement, W.C., Carskadon, M.A., Ley, R. (1973) The prevalence of narcolepsy. *Sleep Res.*, **2**, 147.

33   Yoss, R.E., Daly, D.D. (1960) Narcolepsy in children. *Pediatrics*, **25**, 1025–33.

34   Parkes, J.D., Chen, S.Y., Clift, S.J., Dahlitz, M.J., Dunn, G. (1998) The clinical diagnosis of the narcoleptic syndrome. *J. Sleep. Res.*, 7, 41–52.

35   Yoss, R.E., Daly, D.D. (1957) Criteria for the diagnosis of the narcoleptic syndrome. *Proc. Staff Meet. Mayo Clin.*, **32**, 320–8.

36   Zeman, A., Douglas, N., Aylward, R. (2001) Narcolepsy mistaken for epilepsy. *BMJ*, **322**, 216–18.

37   Aldrich, M.S. (1996) The clinical spectrum of narcolepsy and idiopathic hypersomnia. *Neurology*, **46**, 393–401.

38 Parkes, J.D., Fenton, G., Struthers, G., Curzon, G., Kantamaneni, B.D., Buxton, B.H. *et al.* (1974) Narcolepsy and cataplexy. Clinical features, treatment and cerebrospinal fluid findings. *Q. J. Med.*, **43**, 525–36.

39 Broughton, R., Ghanem, Q., Hishikawa, Y., Sugita, Y., Nevsimalova, S., Roth, B. (1981) Life effects of narcolepsy in 180 patients from North America, Asia and Europe compared to matched controls. *Can. J. Neurol. Sci.*, **8**, 299–304.

40 Godbout, R., Montplaisir, J. (1986) All-day performance variations in normal and narcoleptic subjects. *Sleep*, **9**, 200–4.

41 Kales, A., Soldatos, C.R., Bixler, E.O., Caldwell, A., Cadieux, R.J., Verrechio, J.M. *et al.* (1982) Narcolepsy–cataplexy. II. Psychosocial consequences and associated psychopathology. *Arch. Neurol.*, *39*, 169–71.

42 Beusterien, K.M., Rogers, A.E., Walsleben, J.A., Emsellem, H.A., Reblando, J.A., Wang, L. *et al.* (1999) Health-related quality of life effects of modafinil for treatment of narcolepsy. *Sleep*, 22, 757–65.

43 Daniels, E., King, M.A., Smith, I.E., Shneerson, J.M. (2001) Health-related quality of life in narcolepsy. *J. Sleep Res.*, **10**, 75–81.

44 Findley, L., Unverzagt, M., Guchu, R., Fabrizio, M., Buckner, J., Suratt, P. (1995) Vigilance and automobile accidents in patients with sleep apnea or narcolepsy. *Chest*, **108**, 619–24.

45 George, C.F., Boudreau, A.C., Smiley, A. (1996) Comparison of simulated driving performance in narcolepsy and sleep apnea patients. *Sleep*, **19**, 711–17.

46 Aldrich, M.S., Chervin, R.D., Malow, B.A. (1997) Value of the multiple sleep latency test (MSLT) for the diagnosis of narcolepsy. *Sleep*, **20**, 620–9.

47 Carskadon, M.A., Dement, W.C., Mitler, M.M., Roth, T., Westbrook, P.R., Keenan, S. (1986) Guidelines for the multiple sleep latency test (MSLT): a standard measure of sleepiness. *Sleep*, **9**, 519–24.

48 Ferrans, C.E., Cohen, F.L., Smith, K.M. (1992) The quality of life of persons with narcolepsy, in *Psychosocial Aspects of Narcolepsy*, M. Goswami, C.P. Pollack, F.L. Cohen, M.J. Thorpy, M.B. Cavey (eds), pp. 23–32. New York: Howarth Press.

49 Rosenthal, L.D., Merlotti, L., Young, D.K., Zorick, F.J., Wittig, R.M., Roehrs, T.A. *et al.* (1990) Subjective and polysomnographic characteristics of patients diagnosed with narcolepsy. *Gen. Hosp. Psychiatry*, **12**, 191–7.

50 Rogers, A.E., Aldrich, M.S. (1993) The effect of regularly scheduled naps on sleep attacks and excessive daytime sleepiness associated with narcolepsy. *Nurs. Res.*, **42**, 111–17.

51 Roehrs, T.A., Zorick, F.J., Wittig, R.M., Roth, T. (1986) Dose determinants of rebound insomnia. *Br. J. Clin. Pharmacol.*, **22**, 143–7.

52 Mullington, J., Broughton, R. (1993) Scheduled naps in the management of daytime sleepiness in narcolepsy–cataplexy. *Sleep*, **16**, 444–56.

53 Parkes, J.D., Dahlitz, M. (1993) Amphetamine prescription. *Sleep*, **16**, 201–3.

54 Mitler, M.M., Aldrich, M.S., Koob, G.F., Zarcone, V.P. (1994) Narcolepsy and its treatment with stimulants. ASDA standards of practice. *Sleep*, **17**, 352–71.

55 Mignot, E., Nishino, S., Guilleminault, C., Dement, W.C. (1994) Modafinil binds to the dopamine uptake carrier site with low affinity. *Sleep*, **17**, 436–7.

56 Lin, J.S., Roussel, B., Akaoka, H., Fort, P., Debilly, G., Jouvet, M. (1992) Role of catecholamines in the modafinil and amphetamine induced wakefulness, a comparative pharmacological study in the cat. *Brain Res.*, **591**, 319–26.

57 Besset, A., Chetrit, M., Carlander, B., Billiard, M. (1996) Use of modafinil in the treatment of narcolepsy: a long term follow-up study. *Neurophysiol. Clin.*, **26**, 60–6.

58 Broughton, R.J., Fleming, J.A., George, C.F., Hill, J.D., Kryger, M.H., Moldofsky, H. *et al.* (1997) Randomized, double-blind, placebo-controlled crossover trial of modafinil in the treatment of excessive daytime sleepiness in narcolepsy. *Neurology*, **49**, 444–51.

59 US Modafinil in Narcolepsy Multicenter Study Group. (1998) Randomized trial of modafinil for the treatment of pathological somnolence in narcolepsy. *Ann. Neurol.*, **43**, 88–97.

60 US Modafinil in Narcolepsy Multicenter Study Group. (2000) Randomized trial of modafinil as a treatment for the excessive daytime somnolence of narcolepsy. *Neurology*, **54**, 1166–75.

61 Parkes, J.D., Schachter, M. (1979) Mazindol in the treatment of narcolepsy. *Acta Neurol. Scand.*, **60**, 250–4.

62 Hublin, C., Partinen, M., Heinonen, E.H., Puukka, P., Salmi, T. (1994) Selegiline in the treatment of narcolepsy. *Neurology*, **44**, 2095–101.

63 Lammers, G.J., Arends, J., Declerck, A.C., Ferrari, M.D., Schouwink, G., Troost, J. (1993) Gammahydroxybutyrate and narcolepsy: a double-blind placebo-controlled study. *Sleep*, **16**, 216–20.

64 Mitler, M.M. (1994) Evaluation of treatment with stimulants in narcolepsy. *Sleep*, **17**, S103–6.

65 Guilleminault, C., Carskadon, M., Dement, W.C. (1974) On the treatment of rapid eye movement narcolepsy. *Arch. Neurol.*, **30**, 90–3.

66 Mitler, M.M., Hajdukovic, R. (1991) Relative efficacy of drugs for the treatment of sleepiness in narcolepsy. *Sleep*, **14**, 218–20.

67 Rudd, P. (1995) Clinicians and patients with hypertension: unsettled issues about compliance. *Am. Heart J.*, **130**, 572–9.

68 General Medical Council. (2000) *Confidentiality: Protecting and Providing Information.* London: GMC.

Other causes of sleepiness

Other causes of hypersomnolence may be classified into those causing prolonged and those causing recurrent sleepiness.

Prolonged sleepiness

INSUFFICIENT SLEEP

Being underslept is the most common cause of sleepiness. Sleep requirements vary between individuals but 6.5–8 hours per night appears to be optimal for most. Thirty minutes less sleep per night may make one feel sleepy.[1] Reducing nocturnal sleep time to five hours per night results in subjective sleepiness and impaired mood after one night[2] and objective impairment of vigilance after two nights[2,3] with a progressive decrease in vigilance thereafter up to 60 days.[2,4] The elderly are more sensitive to loss of sleep with more ready impairment of cognitive function.[5]

Clinical features
Most patients present with daytime sleepiness at the normal times – in the afternoon and early evening. Irritability, depression, impaired concentration and decreased vigilance may occur. If the sleep deprivation is work-related, it is common to find that individuals sleep much longer at weekends than during the week. Indeed, the presence of weekend sleep extension is often used to determine whether short sleepers are sleep-depriving themselves mid-week.

Investigation
This is not often required if the history is clear. Sometimes a sleep diary (Chapter 6) may be needed to allow patients to appreciate how little time they are spending in bed.

Treatment
Sleep time should be increased by an hour or more each night. Education about the hazards of sleepiness, particularly when driving, is critical.

IDIOPATHIC HYPERSOMNOLENCE

This is a poorly characterized and understood condition that has also been called essential hypersomnolence or idiopathic central nervous system hypersomnia. It was thought to be a relatively common cause of sleepiness, but the emergence of the obstructive sleep apnoea syndrome and particularly the use of adequate sensors to detect hypopnoeas has resulted in this diagnosis of exclusion becoming much less common. It is now believed to affect around four per 100,000,[6,7] a prevalence one-tenth that of narcolepsy and one-thousandth that of obstructive sleep apnoea/hypopnoea syndrome (OSAHS). Thus many of the earlier series will have contained patients with narcolepsy and OSAHS, making the relevance of the earlier descriptions of the condition limited. It is likely that this diagnosis is still being used to encompass several different disease processes.

Aetiology
Unknown

Epidemiology
Onset is usually between the first and fifth decade with peak onset in the teens. The condition develops over the course of a few weeks or months and tends to persist thereafter, often for life.

Clinical features
Patients experience long periods of daytime drowsiness which significantly impair their performance and quality of life. The drowsiness produces naps which tend to be prolonged, often lasting longer than an hour. These naps are usually unrefreshing. Night sleep duration is often excessively long. In the morning, wakening is difficult and slow and sleep drunkenness may occur.[6,8] It is difficult to awaken the patients and they may be abusive and violent when woken. The combination of the unrefreshing nature of the naps and the potential for abnormal behaviour thereafter sometimes makes patients struggle to avoid napping.

During the periods of drowsiness, patients may develop automatic behaviour during which one- to four-second microsleeps intervene more and more frequently into wakefulness.[9] Patients may find they have unknowingly performed complex and sometimes inappropriate tasks in these episodes, for example driving for several miles in the wrong direction or speaking or writing absolute rubbish. Subjects have no recollection of these events, only awareness of the consequences.

Differential diagnosis

The major conditions which need to be distinguished are OSAHS and narcolepsy, and for further discussion *see* Chapter 5. Essentially, OSAHS can usually be differentiated by the onset in middle age, the presence of loud intermittent snoring and a normal nocturnal sleep duration. Narcolepsy will be confirmed by the co-existence of cataplexy, and suggested by sleep paralysis, sleep-related hallucinations, normal nocturnal sleep duration, sleep disturbance and the low frequency of morning drunkenness.

Diagnosis

Idiopathic hypersomnolence is a diagnosis of exclusion. A 'firm' diagnosis requires normal overnight polysomnography, including demonstration of normal nasal or oesophageal pressure swings[10–12] and/or the absence of recurrent arousals from sleep.[13,14] A multiple sleep latency test (MSLT) should also be performed both to confirm the presence of objective daytime sleepiness and to exclude the presence of sleep onset REM sleeps (SOREMs) suggestive of narcolepsy. On average, patients with idiopathic hypersomnia are less sleepy than those with narcolepsy, with a mean sleep latency on the MSLT of seven minutes in comparison to three minutes in narcoleptic subjects[15] but the ranges overlap. Problems often arise when narcolepsy presents without cataplexy and then the absence of sleep onset REM periods may be helpful.

Treatment

As the cause of this condition is unknown, treatment is symptomatic only. Modification of lifestyle and sleep habits produces little benefit. Planned daytime naps are unhelpful and may result in ensuing confusional episodes. Alcohol, sleep deprivation and shift work should be avoided.

Stimulant drugs are the only agents which have an appreciable effect on the patient's sleepiness. The usual agents used are methylphenidate, mazindol, modafinil or dexamphetamine (*see* Chapter 3 for fuller discussion of these drugs). The usual principles apply, the weakest agent in the lowest effective dose being used while minimizing side-effects.

Useful reviews

- Bassetti, C., Aldrich, M.S. (1997) Idiopathic hypersomnia. A series of 42 patients. *Brain*, **120**, 1423–35.
- Billiard, M., Merle, C., Carlander, B., Ondze, B., Alvarez, D., Besset, A. (1998) Idiopathic hypersomnia. *Psychiatry Clin. Neurosci.*, **52**, 125–9.

PLMD and restless leg syndrome

Periodic limb movements (PLMs) occur every 20–40 seconds during non-REM sleep in some people (Figure 4.1). They are common, occurring in 30 per cent of 50–65-year-olds and nearly 50 per cent of over 65-year-olds.[16] However, more than five PLMs per hour slept is conventionally considered to be pathological[17] and to be diagnostic of the periodic limb movement disorder (PLMD). Despite this, most people with PLMs are asymptomatic.

PLMs are associated with evidence of arousal – albeit sometimes not detectable on EEG.[18] An association is believed to exist between recurrent limb movements and daytime sleepiness but there is no correlation between

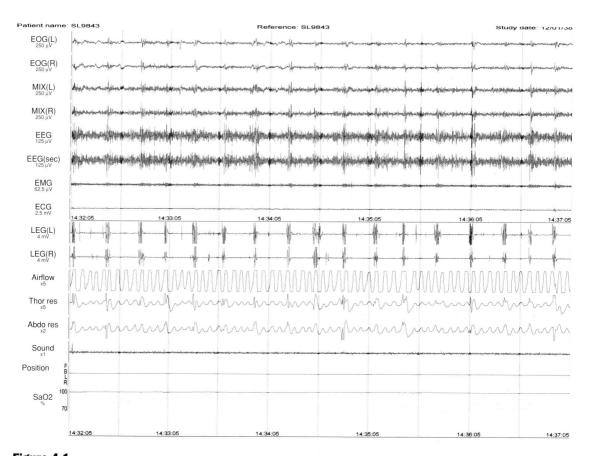

Figure 4.1

Polysomnographic recording of periodic limb movements (PLMs) during sleep with 17 sets of movements over this five-minute period.

PLM frequency and sleepiness across individuals.[18] The situation is further confused as some patients may previously have been mislabelled as having 'PLMD', when they actually had OSAHS[19,20] with their limb movements occurring in association with hypopnoea-induced arousals, but their hypopnoeas may have been missed because inadequate (thermal) sensors[21] were used.

PLMD is associated with restless leg syndrome (RLS), which is characterized by paraesthaesia or dysaesthaesia of the legs, an intense urge to move them and motor restlessness. All the symptoms are worse in the evening or night.[22]

There are placebo-controlled studies showing benefit in patients with RLS from L-dopa[23,24] or pergolide[25] in terms of reducing PLMs and improving subjective sleep quality. However, there are no adequately powered randomized controlled trials investigating the benefits of any therapy in PMLD without restless legs.[26] It is thus questionable whether it is necessary to investigate sleepy individuals for PLMD, unless they have symptoms of RLS, or whether PLMD even exists as a distinct clinical syndrome causing sleepiness.[27] However, conventional wisdom is that patients without an obvious cause for their sleepiness should be investigated for PLMD. These conditions are discussed further in Chapter 8.

OTHER CAUSES OF HYPERSOMNIA

A wide variety of conditions can cause prolonged or temporary, but non-recurrent, sleepiness.

Regular sleep disturbance

Environmental factors may contribute to regular sleep disturbance. For example, new parents often have disturbed sleep for many nights, or weeks, in a row. This often affects the mother more than the father and the parents may develop symptoms due to sleep disruption/deprivation, including sleepiness, depression, irritability and difficulty with making decisions. Similarly, many regular events may disturb sleep, from partner's restlessness or snoring to aircraft or traffic noise.[28]

Phase alteration syndromes and **shift work sleep disorder** need to be considered in sleepy patients and are discussed in Chapter 7.

Alcohol

Evening alcohol disturbs sleep in the later part of the night and can cause sleepiness the next day. These effects seem to decrease with regular alcohol use.[29]

Medications

Daytime sleepiness can result from sedative drugs, such as benzodiazepines and barbituates, and from drugs in which sedation is a side-effect, such as classical antihistamines, tricyclic antidepressants and lipophilic beta-blockers.[30] Sleepiness can also result from sleep disturbance due to use of stimulant drugs too close to bedtime.

Neurological lesions

Tumours and infarcts of the brain can both cause marked sleepiness. This is particularly common in tumours affecting the posterolateral hypothalamus, pineal or upper brainstem and infarcts affecting the paramedian thalamopeduncular area.[31] Head injuries may be followed by sustained sleepiness, usually starting within one year of the injury. This may be associated with headache, memory loss and difficulty concentrating. It can be difficult to determine whether these symptoms have an organic basis. Multiple sclerosis and Wernicke's encephalopathy may also be complicated by sleepiness. Encephalitis lethargica, once a major cause of sleepiness, is now extremely rare.

Trypanosomiasis

Several years after the initial infection in an endemic area, cerebral trypanosomiasis may present with abnormal sleepiness, headache, tremor and choreiform movements. EEG differentiates wakefulness and REM sleep but non-REM is difficult to identify. Treatment is directed at the infection.

Psychogenic

Some people react to stress by increased sleepiness and longer sleep duration. This is usually situational and passes when the stressful situation resolves. In some, the symptoms may be longer term, lasting months or years. Often there is no objective sleepiness on MSLT. Diagnosis depends on the demonstration of psychological problems.

Psychiatric

Major depressive illness and bipolar affective disorders can be associated with significant hypersomnolence. Sometimes the symptoms may be out of keeping with objective measures of sleepiness. Rarely sleepiness can be found in schizophrenia.

Recurrent sleepiness

KLEINE–LEVIN SYNDROME

This rare syndrome is characterized by recurrent attacks of daytime sleepiness associated with bizarre eating and sometimes with hypersexuality.

Aetiology
Unknown. The onset in teenage years[32] and association with disturbance of sleep and sometimes temperature rhythms has lead some to suggest a hypothalamic origin, but this is speculative.

Epidemiology
The condition is rare with only a few hundred cases reported. At least three times as many males as females are affected.[32]

Clinical features
The most marked features are attacks of prolonged sleep and alterations of appetite. During each episode the patient may sleep for more than 20 of the 24 hours. Attacks last from a few days to several weeks with an average of five to seven days. The gap between attacks is variable within and between patients but is often around six months ranging from a month to a year. During attacks the patient may be difficult to rouse to a reasonable level of responsiveness. However, spontaneous awakenings to use the toilet do occur and incontinence is unusual.

Immediately before and during attacks there may be changes in awareness and mood and in cognitive and sexual function. Tearful and disinhibited behaviour may be exhibited suggesting frontal lobe dysfunction. Hypersexuality occurs in perhaps 25 per cent of cases during and immediately after the attacks. This is totally out of keeping with the patient's normal behaviour. Overeating before and during attacks can be extreme with weight gains of up to 10 kg in an attack. Cases occur without co-existing eating or mental disturbance, and indeed this variant may be more common than the classical form of the syndrome.

Attacks are often followed by depression and disgust at the overeating, but sometimes by euphoria and sleeplessness. Occasionally anorexia may occur.

Although Kleine–Levin syndrome was originally reported to be self-limiting, only 20 per cent of 96 subjects followed for a mean of six years had stopped having attacks.[33] Longer follow-up studies are needed.

Differential diagnosis

Other causes of recurrent sleepiness include menstrual associated hypersomnia, hypersomnia secondary to central nervous system (CNS) lesions and psychiatric-associated hypersomnias.

Diagnosis

The clinical presentation may suffice in classic forms of the syndrome. However, all patients will require a neurological history and examination and usually a psychological/psychiatric opinion. Most will require neuroimaging to exclude a CNS lesion. Demonstration of prolonged sleep durations by EEG recordings during attacks can be useful supportive evidence for the diagnosis and excluding the feigning of sleep.

Treatment

Stimulant therapy may reduce the severity of sleep attacks in some patients, but does not prevent attacks. Lithium reduces attacks in some, but not all, cases[34,35] and carbamazepine may also prevent attacks.

OTHER CAUSES OF INTERMITTENT HYPERSOMNIA

Menstrual-related

Rarely, severe sleepiness may recur at the start of the menstrual cycle. This usually commences in adolescence. EEG studies during attacks show prolonged sleep durations.[36] Treatment with the oral contraceptive pill may be effective.[36,37]

CNS lesions

Head injuries, cerebrovascular disease, encephalitis and third ventricular tumours can all cause intermittent attacks of sleepiness.

Psychiatric causes

Intermittent depression can cause recurrent sleepiness.

References

1 Carskadon, M.A., Dement, W.C. (1981) Cumulative effects of sleep restriction on daytime sleepiness. *Psychophysiology*, **18**, 107–13.
2 Dinges, D.F., Pack, F., Williams, K., Gillen, K.A., Powell, J.W., Ott, G.E. *et al.* (1997) Cumulative sleepiness, mood disturbance, and psychomotor vigilance performance decrements during a week of sleep restricted to 4–5 hours per night. *Sleep*, **20**, 267–77.

3   Wilkinson, R.T., Edwards, R.S., Haines, E. (1966) Performance following a night of reduced sleep. *Psychonomic Sci.*, **5**, 472.

4   Webb, W.B., Agnew, H.W. (1974) The effects of a chronic limitation of sleep length. *Psychophysiology*, **11**, 265–74.

5   Webb, W.B. (1985) A further analysis of age and sleep deprivation effects. *Psychophysiology*, **22**, 156–61.

6   Bassetti, C., Aldrich, M.S. (1997) Idiopathic hypersomnia. A series of 42 patients. *Brain*, **120**, 1423–35.

7   Billiard, M., Merle, C., Carlander, B., Ondze, B., Alvarez, D., Besset, A. (1998) Idiopathic hypersomnia. *Psychiatry Clin. Neurosci.*, **52**, 125–9.

8   Roth, B., Nevsimalova, S., Rechtschaffen, A. (1972) Hypersomnia with 'sleep drunkenness'. *Arch. Gen. Psychiatry*, **26**, 456–62.

9   Guilleminault, C., Phillips, R., Dement, W.C. (1975) A syndrome of hypersomnia with automatic behavior. *Electroencephalogr. Clin. Neurophysiol.*, **38**, 403–13.

10   Douglas, N.J. (2000) Upper airway resistance syndrome is not a distinct syndrome. *Am. J. Respir. Crit. Care Med.*, **161**, 1413–15.

11   Rees, K., Kingshott, R.N., Wraith, P.K., Douglas, N.J. (2000) Frequency and significance of increased upper airway resistance during sleep. *Am. J. Respir. Crit. Care Med.*, **162**, 1210–14.

12   Guilleminault, C., Chowdhuri, S. (2000) Upper airway resistance syndrome is a distinct syndrome. *Am. J. Respir. Crit. Care Med.*, **161**, 1412–13.

13   Mathur, R., Douglas, N.J. (1995) Frequency of EEG arousals from nocturnal sleep in normal subjects. *Sleep*, **18**, 330–3.

14   Martin, S.E., Engleman, H.M., Kingshott, R.N., Douglas, N.J. (1997) Microarousals in patients with sleep apnoea/hypopnoea syndrome. *J. Sleep Res.*, **6**, 276–80.

15   van den Hoed, J., Kraemer, H., Guilleminault, C., Zarcone, V.P. Jr, Miles, L.E., Dement, W.C. *et al.* (1981) Disorders of excessive daytime somnolence: polygraphic and clinical data for 100 patients. *Sleep*, **4**, 23–37.

16   Ancoli-Israel, S., Kripke, D.F., Mason, W., Kaplan, O.J. (1985) Sleep apnea and periodic movements in an aging sample. *J. Gerontol.*, **40**, 419–25.

17   Hening, W., Allen, R., Earley, C., Kushida, C., Picchietti, D., Silber, M. (1999) The treatment of restless legs syndrome and periodic limb movement disorder. An American Academy of Sleep Medicine Review. *Sleep*, **22**, 970–99.

18   Winkelman, J.W. (1999) The evoked heart rate response to periodic leg movements of sleep. *Sleep*, **22**, 575–80.

19   Briellmann, R.S., Mathis, J., Bassetti, C., Gugger, M., Hess, C.W.

(1997) Patterns of muscle activity in legs in sleep apnea patients before and during nCPAP therapy. *Eur. Neurol.*, **38**, 113–18.

20 Exar, E.N., Collop, N.A. (2001) The association of upper airway resistance with periodic limb movements. *Sleep*, **24**, 188–92.

21 American Sleep Disorders Association. (1999) Sleep-related breathing disorders in adults: recommendations for syndrome definition and measurement techniques in clinical research. The Report of an American Academy of Sleep Medicine Task Force. *Sleep*, **22**, 667–89.

22 Chesson, A.L. Jr, Wise, M., Davila, D., Johnson, S., Littner, M., Anderson, W.M. *et al.* (1999) Practice parameters for the treatment of restless legs syndrome and periodic limb movement disorder. An American Academy of Sleep Medicine Report. Standards of Practice Committee of the American Academy of Sleep Medicine. *Sleep*, **22**, 961–8.

23 Benes, H., Kurella, B., Kummer, J., Kazenwadel, J., Selzer, R., Kohnen, R. (1999) Rapid onset of action of levodopa in restless legs syndrome: a double-blind, randomized, multicenter, crossover trial. *Sleep*, **22**, 1073–81.

24 Trenkwalder, C., Stiasny, K., Pollmacher, T., Wetter, T., Schwarz, J., Kohnen, R. *et al.* (1995) L-dopa therapy of uremic and idiopathic restless legs syndrome: a double-blind, crossover trial. *Sleep*, **18**, 681–8.

25 Wetter, T.C., Stiasny, K., Winkelmann, J., Buhlinger, A., Brandenburg, U., Penzel, T. *et al.* (1999) A randomized controlled study of pergolide in patients with restless legs syndrome. *Neurology*, **52**, 944–50.

26 Hening ,W., Allen, R., Earley, C., Kushida, C., Picchietti, D., Silber, M. (1999) The treatment of restless legs syndrome and periodic limb movement disorder. An American Academy of Sleep Medicine Review. *Sleep*, **22**, 970–99.

27 Nicolas, A., Lesperance, P., Montplaisir, J. (1998) Is excessive daytime sleepiness with periodic leg movements during sleep a specific diagnostic category? *Eur. Neurol.*, **40**, 22–6.

28 Horne, J.A., Pankhurst, F.L., Reyner, L.A., Hume, K., Diamond, I.D. (1994) A field study of sleep disturbance: effects of aircraft noise and other factors on 5,742 nights of actimetrically monitored sleep in a large subject sample. *Sleep*, **17**, 146–59.

29 Rundell, O.H., Lester, B.K., Griffiths, W.J., Williams, H.L. (1972) Alcohol and sleep in young adults. *Psychopharmacologia*, **26**, 201–18.

30 Kostis, J.B., Rosen, R.C. (1987) Central nervous system effects of beta-adrenergic-blocking drugs: the role of ancillary properties. *Circulation*, **75**, 204–12.

31 Castaigne, P., Lhermitte, F., Buge, A., Escourolle, R., Hauw, J.J., Lyon-Caen, O. (1981) Paramedian thalamic and midbrain infarct: clinical and neuropathological study. *Ann. Neurol.*, **10**, 127–48.

32 Kesler, A., Gadoth, N., Vainstein, G., Peled, R., Lavie, P. (2000) Kleine Levin syndrome (KLS) in young females. *Sleep*, **23**, 563–7.

33 Billiard, M. (1980) The Kleine–Levin syndrome, in W.P. Koella (ed). *Sleep*, pp. 436–43. Basel: Karger.

34 Abe, K. (1977) Lithium prophylaxis of periodic hypersomnia. *Br. J. Psychiatry*, **130**, 312–13.

35 Hart, E.J. (1985) Kleine–Levin syndrome: normal CSF monoamines and response to lithium therapy. *Neurology*, **35**, 1395–6.

36 Billiard, M., Guilleminault, C., Dement, W.C. (1975) A menstruation-linked periodic hypersomnia. Kleine–Levin syndrome or new clinical entity? *Neurology*, **25**, 436–43.

37 Sachs, C., Persson, H.E., Hagenfeldt, K. (1982) Menstruation-related periodic hypersomnia: a case study with successful treatment. *Neurology*, **32**, 1376–9.

Investigating the sleepy patient

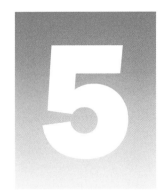

Determining the cause of daytime sleepiness is one of the commonest tasks for physicians in sleep medicine. Often the cause is obvious once an appropriate history has been taken, although further investigation is usually required unless sleep deprivation or shift work is the cause. However, sometimes the diagnosis may still be unclear despite extensive investigation, in which case clinical skill and judgement – and occasionally trial and error – may be the deciding factors between successful treatment and continued impairment of quality of life for patients and their families.

History

Sleepy patients and their partners or parents should all be sent questionnaires about sleep habits and key symptoms to complete before the initial consultation. This should include at least the topics covered in Table 5.1.

Examination

Few features on examination can point to a definite diagnosis unless the physician witnesses a cataplectic attack. The observation of snoring and apnoeas in a sleeping patient is suggestive but not diagnostic. Similarly, obesity, increased neck girth, nasal or pharyngeal obstruction, a receding jaw and hypertension may be helpful pointers to obstructive sleep apnoea/hypopnoea syndrome (OSAHS).

Need for further investigation

Patients with a clear history of inadequate sleep duration or sleep disruption due to shift work may need no further investigation before a firm diagnosis is made unless there are pointers (Table 5.2) to other sleep problems. Most

Table 5.1

Components of a sleep questionnaire for sleepy patients

Sleep duration and quality
  Normal bed or lights out time working days and weekends
  Usual time to fall asleep
  Time of final awakening working days and weekends
  Number and duration of wakenings throughout the night
  Cause of nocturnal wakenings
Daytime naps
Shift working
  Precise timing and pattern of shifts
Duration of symptoms
  Age at onset
  Progression of symptoms
  Severity of symptoms
Associated symptoms
  Snoring, including frequency, severity and positionality
  Witnessed apnoeas
  Nocturnal choking
  Unrefreshing sleep
  Cataplexy
  Hypnogogic hallucinations
  Sleep paralysis
  Witnessed recurrent limb movements during sleep
Predisposing factors
  Weight gain
  Quantity of alcohol consumed
  Family history of sleep apnoea or narcolepsy
  Psychological or psychiatric illness
  Potentially sedating or stimulant drugs, including caffeine
Severity of sleepiness
  Epworth[1] (see page 47) or other sleepiness scale
  Frequency and consequences of sleepiness: driving; at work; in
embarrassing social situations
  Effect on work performance and ability to concentrate

other patients will require further investigation as the response to the questions are likely to suggest, rather than prove, a diagnosis.

It has been argued that patients with a clear history of sleepiness plus cataplexy require no further investigation. I believe this is rarely if ever the case. Narcolepsy is a life-long illness and a life-long label to attach to patients, with major potential effects on their work, ability to drive and quality of life. Thus it is essential to ensure that the label is only applied correctly. In addition, sometimes there may be concern that patients are

	OSAHS	Narcolepsy	IHS
Age of onset (years)	35–60	10–30	10–30
Night sleep			
Duration	Normal	Normal	Long
Awakenings	Occasional	Frequent	Rare
Snoring	Yes	Occasional	Occasional
Morning drunkenness	Occasional	Occasional	Common
Day naps			
Frequency	Usually few	Many	Few
Time of day	Afternoon/evening	Afternoon/evening	Morning
Duration	<1 hour	<1 hour	>1 hour

Features suggesting obstructive sleep apnoea/hypopnoea syndrome (OSAHS), narcolepsy or idiopathic hypersomnolence (IHS).

Table 5.2
Clinical pointers in the sleepy patient

faking their symptoms in order to obtain access to stimulant drugs or for psychological reasons. Most sleep centres have experience of such patients, who often present with a full house of narcoleptic symptoms and can only be detected by negative investigations, particularly a normal multiple sleep latency test (MSLT). Although I believe this fear can be overplayed, anxieties of medical and allied staff, and sometimes of family and friends, can be allayed by simple investigations which allow a definitive diagnosis to be made.

Investigations

Clinical investigation of patients with sleepiness may involve either investigation of abnormalities during sleep – usually performed overnight – or investigation of the magnitude of daytime sleepiness.

INVESTIGATION DURING SLEEP

Studies of patterns of sleep, breathing and/or movements during sleep may be performed with any degree of complexity from one to sometimes 30 channels of information being recorded during part or all of a night's sleep. Conventionally, these are termed either 'full polysomnography' where sleep is recorded from an adequate number of electro-physiological signals as well as breathing and limb movements. On the other hand, limited-sleep studies usually record breathing but less or no information about sleep duration and quality. The complexity of both approaches can vary markedly but the types of signals often recorded are listed below.

Polysomnography

Sleep from:

- Electro-encephalogram – usually at least two leads, one central, one frontal.
- Electromyography – usually sub-mental.
- Electro-oculography.

Respiratory signals (*see* Chapter 2):

- 'Airflow' from nasal pressure, nasal temperature, expired CO_2 or, rarely, by pneumotach with a facemask.
- 'Ventilation' from thoraco-abdominal movement or nasal pressure.
- Oxygenation from an oximeter.
- Carbon dioxide from a transcutaneous capnometer.
- Evidence of airflow obstruction from nasal or oesophageal pressure sensors or derived from other indirect signals such as pulse transit time (PTT).

Leg movements from electromyography or piezo-electric detectors.

Other signals:

- ECG.
- Pulse rate.
- Posture.
- Oesophageal pH.
- Sound or objective snoring intensity.
- Video recording.

For routine polysomnography the montage should include at least:

- For sleep staging and arousals: two EEGs, EOG and EMG.
- Respiratory: nasal pressure; thoraco-abdominal movement; oximeter.
- Other: EMG or piezo-electric leg movement; posture; snoring noise; ECG.

This montage allows some built-in redundancy in case a sensor fails, for example there are two EEG leads and three breathing pattern monitors.

The clinical value of performing polysomnography on all patients with daytime sleepiness has been questioned.[2] In a prospective study of 200 patients with possible OSAHS, the overnight polysomnography records were analysed to determine which signals contributed to a diagnosis being made. The conclusion was that the respiratory variables – thoraco-abdominal movement and oximetry – and the leg movement sensors were helpful but the neurophysiological signals did not contribute significantly to the diagnosis in these patients. Thus sleep studies which did not record sleep might be diagnostically helpful and cheaper.

Polysomnography usually requires about 30–60 minutes' set-up time before sleep and about 30 minutes' detachment time in the morning. Thus staff will need to be available for at least 10 hours per night. The study will take one to four hours to analyse. The actual cost of polysomnography will depend on the staffing levels used, the number of studies being performed and the cost of the premises and equipment. As a guide, our costs are approximately £250/patient per night (US $350 or Euro 400/patient per night).

Limited-sleep studies

These may theoretically use any cut-down mixture of the above signals, recording from one to many variables. Usually, they focus on respiratory signals often with an indirect measure of arousal as well. Common combinations are airflow, thoraco-abdominal movement, oximetry and heart rate with some adding snoring and indirect evidence of episodes of airflow obstruction. Several different systems are available and some have been adequately validated.[3-5] However, this field is changing so fast that no book can usefully advocate a best buy system.

Limited-sleep studies can often be done in the home with patients applying the sensors themselves after instruction from sleep technicians. A written instruction sheet should also be provided. Home studies can be used to unequivocally diagnose both OSAHS (Figure 5.1) and periodic limb movement disorder (PLMD) (Figure 5.2) while saving the costs both of the accommodation in the sleep centre and the attendant staff. Indeed, in our hands such studies cost approximately 22 per cent of a polysomnography.

However, this has to set against a possible decrease in diagnostic certainty as limited studies do not allow assessment of sleep. Thus some respiratory events occurring during wakefulness will be scored[4] and patients who totally fail to sleep will have negative studies – although this is rare in OSAHS. In reality the financial analysis of the use of limited-sleep studies will need to be examined by each sleep centre depending on the costs, the geographical catchment area served, the equipment, the diagnostic algorithm used and the extent 'split-night' CPAP titration studies are used. Into the calculation needs to be factored the costs of both limited and polysomnography studies in the percentage of patients who require both studies. However, by use of this approach (Figure 5.3) we have been able to reduce costs by 22 per cent

Figure 5.1
Limited-sleep study recordings of OSAHS showing from above-leg EMG, chest movement, flow and oxygen saturation over a five-minute period.

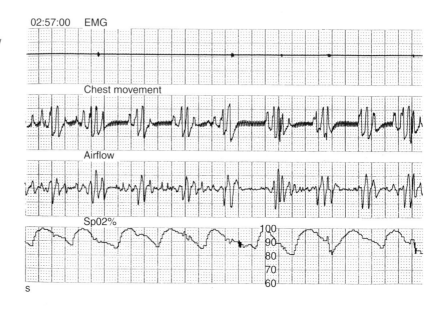

Limited sleep study in OSAHS

Figure 5.2
Limited-sleep study showing recurrent periodic leg movements (PLMs). Montage as Figure 5.1.

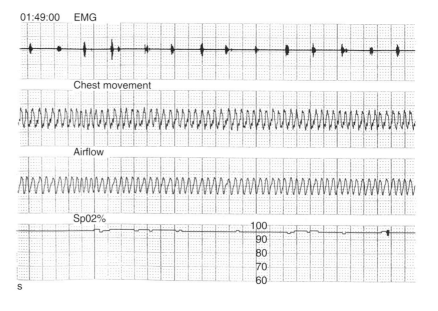

Limited sleep study in PLMD

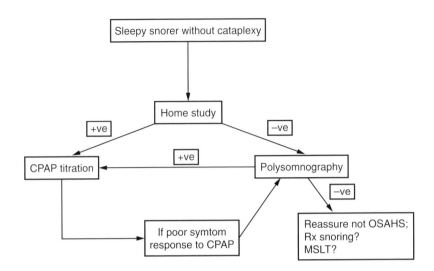

Figure 5.3
Flow diagram of investigation of patients with possible OSAHS.

and speed up diagnosis by a median of 62 per cent without affecting subsequent CPAP use.[5]

Considerable attention has been paid to the use of oximetry alone studies to diagnose OSAHS, and widely divergent conclusions have been reached.[2,6–10] It is difficult to reconcile these views. A possible explanation is that those studies which defined hypopnoeas as requiring coincident desaturation, not surprisingly found that oximetry alone was useful,[6,9,10] whereas those that could diagnose hypopnoeas in the absence of desaturation found a that approximately one-third of cases of OSAHS were missed by oximetry alone.[2,8]

There is no doubt that a trained observer can confidently diagnose OSAHS from positive oximetry traces,[2] but the problem is that false negatives are common and a normal oximetry trace does not exclude severe OSAHS which will respond well to treatment. Indeed, younger and thinner OSAHS patients often do not desaturate despite frequent apnoeas and hypopnoeas and it is unacceptable to fail to diagnose such patients. In my view there is no role for oximetry alone studies as they cannot exclude the diagnosis of OSAHS and they add the risk of false negative studies unless no other equipment is available. A much better option is to perform a limited study with respiratory breathing pattern monitoring included and the equipment costs are not much greater. Theoretically, it may be possible to derive indices computed from oximetry traces which contribute usefully to the diagnosis of OSAHS,[7,8,10] but these would seem to be best used in conjunction with other respiratory variables.

MULTIPLE SLEEP LATENCY TESTING

MSLTs are one way of documenting objective sleepiness. Patients are put to bed in a darkened room and the time they take to go to sleep on five naps at two-hour intervals is documented electroencephalographically. Classically, an MSLT score of less than five minutes has been regarded as abnormal[11] and two or more episodes of REM sleep within 15 minutes of sleep onset diagnostic of narcolepsy.[12] However, neither of these assumptions are firm.

The limitations of MSLTs include the fact that normal values have not been adequately defined. In 77 middle-aged control subjects from a community sample, the mean MSLT was 15 minutes (standard deviation (SD) four minutes).[13] In a group of 139 volunteers mean MSLT was 10 minutes (SD five minutes),[14] the greater sleepiness perhaps reflecting response bias, as the subjects had responded to an advertisement for research volunteers for a sleep centre. Mean MSLT was 11 minutes in 130 normal subjects aged 18–29 years and 12.5 minutes in 47 normal subjects aged 30–80 years,[15] although again, these were responding to a request to volunteer for studies in a sleep centre.

A mean MSLT score of less than five or eight minutes is often used to define the pathological sleepiness of narcolepsy.[16] By use of the data of Levine[15] approximately 12 per cent of subjects aged 18–29 years and 10 per cent of those aged 30–80 years had mean MSLTs of five minutes or less, and 40 per cent of subjects aged 18–29 years and 30 per cent of subjects aged 30–80 years had mean MSLTs of eight minutess or less.

In narcolepsy, short sleep latencies are common but not universal even in the presence of cataplexy (Table 5.3). Although there is a need to obtain larger studies of community normals, these data indicate serious limitations to use of these MSLT cuts on their own to define sleepiness or narcolepsy.

Second, the other MSLT criterion used to define narcolepsy is the presence of two or more episodes of sleep onset REM sleep (SOREM), defined as REM sleep within 15 minutes of sleep onset (Table 5.4), which has been reported in 74 per cent of 106 narcoleptic subjects with cataplexy and 91 per

Table 5.3
Mean sleep latencies (SL) in normal subjects and patients with narcolepsy with and without cataplexy

	Mean SL ≤ 5 min	Mean SL ≤ 8 min
Normal subjects aged 18–29 years[15]	12%	40%
Normal subjects aged 30–80 years[15]	10%	30%
Narcolepsy + cataplexy[16]	87%	93%
Narcolepsy – cataplexy[16]	81%	97%

cent of 64 narcoleptic subjects without cataplexy.[16] However, the prevalence of SOREM in the community and in other sleep disorders is less well-documented. Bishop *et al.*[14] found that 17 per cent of their 139 'normal' volunteers had two or more episodes of SOREM during their MSLTs and these subjects denied sleepiness and reported normal nocturnal sleeping habits. Chervin and Aldrich[17] found that five per cent of patients with sleep apnoea/hypopnoea syndrome had two or more SOREMs, and in another paper, reported SOREMs in seven per cent of patients with other non-narcoleptic sleep disorders.[16]

Narcolepsy
Sleep apnoea/hypopnoea syndrome
Sleep deprivation
REM sleep deprivation
Major depression
Drug withdrawal
Alcoholism

Table 5.4
Causes of sleep onset REM sleep[18]

Usually, the MSLT is used to define narcolepsy by a combination of a short sleep latency with the presence of SOREMs.[19] However, even this approach has limitations which must be recognized. First, only 71 per cent of narcoleptic patients with cataplexy have a mean sleep latency of less than eight minutes and two or more SOREMs on initial MSLT, and even after repeated MSLTs, this did not rise above 80 per cent.[16] Second, approximately four per cent of patients with other sleep disorders[16] and around 12 per cent of Bishop's 'normal' subjects[14] also fulfilled these dual criteria. Thus there are no criteria on MSLTs which are **diagnostic** of narcolepsy, at best the results can be supportive of the diagnosis.

Other factors which may affect the MSLT result include activity prior to performing the test which can have a profound effect on the result, a five-minute walk doubling the mean sleep latency compared to 15 minutes watching television.[20] Patient motivation can also influence the result, financial inducements being shown to speed sleep onset.[21]

Despite all these reservations the MSLT can be clinically useful as supporting evidence for a diagnosis or as an excluder of severe sleepiness. However, the limitations of the test should always be remembered.

Conventionally, an MSLT follows overnight polysomnography.[11] However, if the patient does not snore the only point of doing overnight polysomnography is to ensure adequate sleep duration the previous night, and it is doubtful whether the cost of polysomnography is justified to ensure this. Sleeping the previous night at home does not seem to alter sleep latency.[22] Our practice is to let patients sleep at home but to monitor sleep duration using actigraphy. However, further data on the effect this may have on MSLT results is needed before this is adopted as a widespread practice.

MAINTENANCE OF WAKEFULNESS TEST

Whereas the MSLT measures the ability to fall asleep, the problem for sleepy patients is the opposite, namely their inability to keep themselves awake. This can be measured by placing patients in a soporific environment and measuring how long they can resist sleep. This maintenance of wakefulness test (MWT) is carried out with patients seated in a room with dimmed lighting while recording the EEG, EMG and EOG. The test determines whether patients fall asleep on each of four or five naps at two-hour intervals through the day and the time until sleep onset in each case.[23,24]

This test has advantages over the MSLT in that it measure the clinically troubling phenomenon but normal ranges are even less well-standardized. In addition, it does not allow assessment of SOREMs as the test is terminated after 20 minutes, irrespective of sleep onset[24] and even if extended for up to 10 minutes of sleep, one study found that SOREMs were not markedly more common in narcolepsy compared with OSAHS.[25] The test is used in some centres to determine whether individuals are likely to keep awake while driving, but there is no evidence that the results on a single day relate to accident rate. The MWT does reflect improvements with therapy both in OSAHS[26] and narcolepsy.[27,28]

The 'Osler test' is a variant of the MWT which uses the failure of patients to respond to a flashing light rather than the EEG to measure sleep onset.[29] This behavioural test is simpler to perform but is less objective and theoretically open to abuse by patients if they wish to be labelled sleepy. It can reflect improvements with therapy in OSAHS.[30]

Protocol for investigating sleepy patients

'Sleepy' is defined for this section as individuals with a normal nocturnal sleep duration who have:

- Pulled off the road twice in the past year because of sleepiness.
- Unexplained sleepiness impairing work.
- An Epworth sleepiness scale score of more than 11.

The diagnostic pathway will depend on what is the most likely cause.

PROBABLE OSAHS

Sleepy patients with a history of snoring will usually be investigated by a limited sleep study carried out in their homes. If that is unequivocally positive, the patient is diagnosed as having OSAHS and therapy is organized. However, a negative or equivocal study in a sleepy individual **must** result in further investigation, usually overnight polysomnography.

At present we use an Edentrace 2 (Mallinckrodt, St Louis, Missouri) or Embletta (ResMed, San Diego, California) device for home studies. If a sleepy patient has more than 25 apnoeas plus hypopnoeas per hour in bed[5] then it is regarded as unequivocally positive for OSAHS.

PATIENTS WITH PROBABLE NARCOLEPSY

Those who have a story of cataplexy plus sleepiness are studied principally by MSLT. In this group of patients a mean sleep latency of less than eight minutes with at least one SOREMs would be regarded as diagnostic.

In patients who have possible narcolepsy without cataplexy, the diagnostic criteria for narcolepsy should, I believe, be more strict. Thus we perform polysomnography on these patients – to exclude OSAHS and PLMD – and then an MSLT. Those with a normal polysomnography and a mean sleep latency of less than eight minutes with two SOREMs – and no other reasons for SOREMs (*see* page 143) – may be diagnosed as having narcolepsy without cataplexy.

PATIENTS WITH SLEEPINESS BUT NO SNORING OR CATAPLEXY

If these patients have features of depression a psychological or psychiatric opinion may be the initial step. If this is not the case, these patients may require polysomnography followed by an MSLT to both document any sleep-related problem and the extent of sleepiness. Patients who have a normal overnight polysomnography and a mean sleep latency of:

- More than 10 minutes are reassured and discharged unless there are major concerns about their safety driving.
- Five to 10 minutes will need investigations tailored to their clinical problem. If their sleepiness is interfering with work, driving or quality of life then further investigation will usually be warranted, including a repeat MSLT.
- Less than five minutes, whose sleepiness is interfering with work, driving or quality of life will usually require therapy, often with stimulants, and

the need to investigate further will depend on factors such as the quality of the sleep and the recording on the polysomnography and whether there were SOREMs on the MSLT. With a definitely normal polysomnography and in the absence of major psychological/psychiatric illness the occurrence of two SOREMs in this group makes a diagnosis of cataplexy negative narcolepsy reasonable. The absence of SOREMs and a suggestive story would lead to a diagnosis of idiopathic hypersomnolence (IHS).

Patients with history of restless leg syndrome plus sleepiness will have overnight polysomnography to confirm the diagnosis of PLMD before treatment is commenced.

Patients having MSLTs or reporting persisting sleepiness despite normal polysomnography will have unannounced urine drug screens to detect undeclared sedative or stimulant use. The value of this needs testing but anecdotally we and others have found some surprising cases of unsuspected drug-induced sedation.

If drug screen is negative and reported sleepiness severe I perform two weeks of home actigraphy to document sleep durations followed by an MSLT. If nocturnal sleep duration is more than 6.5 hours, a daytime sleep latency of less than eight minutes will result in a trial of therapy; if sleep latency is more than 10 minutes psychological or psychiatric assessment will be discussed.

Episodic sleepiness – where possible, I perform an MSLT during a sleepy episode to document objective sleepiness.

References

1 Johns, M.W. (1991) A new method for measuring daytime sleepiness: the Epworth sleepiness scale. *Sleep*, **14**, 540–5.

2 Douglas, N.J., Thomas, S., Jan, M.A. (1992) Clinical value of polysomnography. *Lancet*, **339**, 347–50.

3 Bradley, P.A., Mortimore, I.L., Douglas, N.J. (1995) Comparison of polysomnography with ResCare Autoset in the diagnosis of the sleep apnoea/hypopnoea syndrome. *Thorax*, **50**, 1201–3.

4 Rees, K., Wraith, P.K., Berthon-Jones, M., Douglas, N.J. (1998) Detection of apnoeas, hypopnoeas and arousals by the AutoSet in the sleep apnoea/hypopnoea syndrome. *Eur. Respir. J.*, **12**, 7649.

5 Whittle, A.T., Finch, S.P., Mortimore, I.L., Mackay, T.W., Douglas, N.J. (1997) Use of home sleep studies for diagnosis of the sleep apnoea/hypopnoea syndrome. *Thorax*, **52**, 1068–73.

6   Series, F., Marc, I., Cormier, Y., La Forge, J. (1993) Utility of nocturnal home oximetry for case finding in patients with suspected sleep apnea hypopnea syndrome. *Ann. Intern. Med.*, **119**, 449–53.

7   Levy, P., Pepin, J.L., Deschaux-Blanc, C., Paramelle, B., Brambilla, C. (1996) Accuracy of oximetry for detection of respiratory disturbances in sleep apnea syndrome. *Chest*, **109**, 395–9.

8   Ryan, P.J., Hilton, M.F., Boldy, D.A., Evans, A., Bradbury, S., Sapiano, S. *et al.* (1995) Validation of British Thoracic Society guidelines for the diagnosis of the sleep apnoea/hypopnoea syndrome: can polysomnography be avoided? *Thorax*, **50**, 972–5.

9   Chiner, E., Signes-Costa, J., Arriero, J.M., Marco, J., Fuentes, I., Sergado, A. (1999) Nocturnal oximetry for the diagnosis of the sleep apnoea hypopnoea syndrome: a method to reduce the number of polysomnographies? *Thorax*, **54**, 968–71.

10 Vazquez, J.C., Tsai, W.H., Flemons, W.W., Masuda, A., Brant, R., Hajduk, E. *et al.* (2000) Automated analysis of digital oximetry in the diagnosis of obstructive sleep apnoea. *Thorax*, **55**, 302–7.

11 Carskadon, M.A., Dement, W.C., Mitler, M.M., Roth, T., Westbrook, P.R., Keenan, S. (1986) Guidelines for the multiple sleep latency test (MSLT): a standard measure of sleepiness. *Sleep*, **9**, 519–24.

12 Mitler, M.M., Van den, H.J., Carskadon, M.A., Richardson, G., Park, R., Guilleminault, C. *et al.* (1979) REM sleep episodes during the Multiple Sleep Latency Test in narcoleptic patients. *Electroencephalogr. Clin. Neurophysiol.*, **46**, 479–81.

13 Kronholm, E., Hyyppa, M.T., Alanen, E., Halonen, J.P., Partinen, M. (1995) What does the multiple sleep latency test measure in a community sample? *Sleep*, **18**, 827–35.

14 Bishop, C., Rosenthal, L., Helmus, T., Roehrs, T., Roth, T. (1996) The frequency of multiple sleep onset REM periods among subjects with no excessive daytime sleepiness. *Sleep*, **19**, 727–30.

15 Levine, B., Roehrs, T., Zorick, F., Roth, T. (1988) Daytime sleepiness in young adults. *Sleep*, **11**, 39–46.

16 Aldrich, M.S., Chervin, R.D., Malow, B.A. (1997) Value of the multiple sleep latency test (MSLT) for the diagnosis of narcolepsy. *Sleep*, **20**, 620–9.

17 Chervin, R.D., Aldrich, M.S. (2000) Sleep onset REM periods during multiple sleep latency tests in patients evaluated for sleep apnea. *Am. J. Respir. Crit. Care Med.*, **161**, 426–31.

18 Association of Sleep Disorders Centers. (1979) Diagnostic classification of sleep and arousal disorders. *Sleep*, **2**, 1–154.

19 Harsh, J., Peszka, J., Hartwig, G., Mitler, M. (2000) Night-time sleep and daytime sleepiness in narcolepsy. *J. Sleep Res.*, **9**, 309–16.

20 Bonnet, M.H., Arand, D.L. (1998) Sleepiness as measured by modified

multiple sleep latency testing varies as a function of preceding activity. *Sleep*, **21**, 477–83.

21 Harrison, Y., Bright, V., Horne, J.A. (1996) Can normal subjects be motivated to fall asleep faster? *Physiol. Behav.*, **60**, 681–4.

22 Kingshott, R.N., Douglas, N.J. (2000) The effect of in laboratory polysomnography on sleep and objective daytime sleepiness. *Sleep*, **23**, 1109–13.

23 Mitler, M.M., Gujavarty, K.S., Browman, C.P. (1982) Maintenance of wakefulness test: a polysomnographic technique for evaluation treatment efficacy in patients with excessive somnolence. *Electroencephalogr. Clin. Neurophysiol.*, **53**, 658–61.

24 Mitler, M.M., Walsleben, J., Sangal, R.B., Hirshkowitz, M. (1998) Sleep latency on the maintenance of wakefulness test (MWT) for 530 patients with narcolepsy while free of psychoactive drugs. *Electroencephalogr. Clin. Neurophysiol.*, **107**, 33–8.

25 Browman, C.P., Gujavarty, K.S., Sampson, M.G., Mitler, M.M. (1983) REM sleep episodes during the maintenance of wakefulness test in patients with sleep apnea syndrome and patients with narcolepsy. *Sleep*, **6**, 23–8.

26 Poceta, J.S., Timms, R.M., Jeong, D.U., Ho, S.L., Erman, M.K., Mitler, M.M. (1992) Maintenance of wakefulness test in obstructive sleep apnea syndrome. *Chest*, **101**, 893–7.

27 US Modafinil in Narcolepsy Multicenter Study Group. (1998) Randomized trial of modafinil for the treatment of pathological somnolence in narcolepsy. *Ann. Neurol.*, **43**, 88–97.

28 US Modafinil in Narcolepsy Multicenter Study Group. (2000) Randomized trial of modafinil as a treatment for the excessive daytime somnolence of narcolepsy. *Neurology*, **54**, 1166–75.

29 Bennett, L.S., Stradling, J.R., Davies, R.J. (1997) A behavioural test to assess daytime sleepiness in obstructive sleep apnoea. *J. Sleep. Res.*, **6**, 142–5.

30 Jenkinson, C., Davies, R.J., Mullins, R., Stradling, J.R. (1999) Comparison of therapeutic and subtherapeutic nasal continuous positive airway pressure for obstructive sleep apnoea: a randomised prospective parallel trial. *Lancet*, **353**, 2100–5.

Insomnia

Definition

Although the word is derived from the Latin for '**no sleep**', insomnia is not defined as absence of sleep nor as a short sleep duration, and normal subjects vary greatly in their sleep requirements. Insomnia is defined as the subjective complaint of insufficient, inadequate or non-restorative sleep.

This definition results in several difficulties for clinicians. First, it is the patient whose opinion determines the use of the diagnostic label. Second, as no laboratory investigation has a close relationship to symptoms, the response to therapy cannot be adequately assessed objectively. Third, patients with insomnia are heterogeneous making the application of clinical trials' results to individual patients difficult.

Aetiology and classification

Patients with a very wide range of situational, psychological, psychiatric and medical conditions can present with insomnia. These may be classified in a variety of ways. This book will follow the major division into short- and long-term insomnia and will consider the numerous different causes under each heading.

Another classification which is sometimes diagnostically helpful is by the time in the sleep process when problems are experienced. Thus, those having difficulty getting to sleep at the beginning of the night – sleep initiation insomnia – may have phase delay syndrome or anxiety. Sleep maintenance insomnia, with difficulty remaining asleep, is common with sleep apnoea/hypopnoea syndrome, periodic limb movement disorder (PLMD), alcohol or caffeine. Early morning wakening insomnia may suggest depression or phase advance syndrome.

Epidemiology

Several surveys have suggested that about a third of Americans reported some insomnia in the past year, with 9–17 per cent stating this was a significant problem.[1-3] Similar prevalences have been reported from other countries.[4] A consistent finding is that insomnia is more common in women and increases with age.

COSTS OF INSOMNIA

The high prevalence is associated with high costs. The estimated costs of drugs used for insomnia in the USA in 1995 was $2 billion, half on prescription and half on over the counter (OTC) drugs.[5] Non-drug healthcare costs were estimated at $12 billion – $11 billion due to nursing home costs – giving a total cost of insomnia of $14 billion per annum. In France, with a population of 22 per cent of the US population, the non-nursing home costs were estimated at US $2 billion.[6] Combining these US and French estimates gives an approximate cost of US $46 million/million population per year.

Clinical features

The defining feature is impaired subjective sleep quality. This may be described in many different ways including difficulty initiating sleep, difficulty maintaining sleep thereafter or non-restorative sleep. These may be the only symptoms, but many will also complain of daytime fatigue causing difficulty accomplishing tasks and impaired concentration and memory. However, there is no evidence of daytime sleepiness in this condition, neither subjective[7] nor objective using the multiple sleep latency test.[8-11] There is also no good evidence of impaired daytime cognitive function.[7,11]

Nevertheless, insomniacs report twice normal rates of motor vehicle accidents.[4,12] Insomniacs are also more likely to report that they suffer from ill health and that illness interferes with their work. About half those complaining of insomnia will have a co-existing psychological disorder such as anxiety, depression or alcohol problems.[4] Many insomniacs will receive treatment with hypnotics and the side-effects of these may also contribute to their daytime symptoms.

SHORT-TERM INSOMNIA

Transient insomnia occurs in individuals who are normally good sleepers. This is caused by problems in the sleeping environment, psychological stress, drug initiation or withdrawal or disruption of the normal circadian sleep schedule.

Stress-related insomnia

Anxieties about life situations commonly interfere with sleep quality. The start of the patient's sleep difficulties coincides with an identifiable stressor. This may be related to any aspect of daily life, including relationships, family, work or money. Bereavement commonly interferes with sleep. In contrast, some people find that euphoria and anticipation of pleasant events causes them to sleep poorly. Cross-sectional questionnaire studies show a poor correlation between stress levels and self-reported sleep disturbance,[13] although this may partly reflect differences between stress levels at the time insomnia started and those subsequently when stress was assessed.

Treatment hinges on education and support. The cornerstone of therapy is reassurance that the symptoms are a normal reaction and will subside as the precipitating event recedes. In most situations, sleep will return to normal within a few weeks. Sufferers should also be helped to understand that daytime naps and extended time in bed at night are contraindicated. Both will interfere with normal circadian rhythms and decrease nocturnal sleepiness, and thus delay the resumption of normal nocturnal sleep patterns. In some acute situations, such as bereavement, a brief course of a short-acting hypnotic may be necessary, but, if so, the lowest effective dose should be used for the shortest possible time.

Expectation

On-call workers sleep poorly whether or not they are disturbed that night.[14] Anecdotally, the same seems to be true of mothers of infants who often cry at night. This expectation of poor sleep may also be a factor in the impaired sleep quality found after withdrawal of hypnotics that have been used long-term. Explanation and support are the most appropriate components of management if the situation cannot be avoided.

Problems in the sleeping environment

Strange location

Most people are familiar with difficulties sleeping in a strange bedroom. This is confirmed in sleep laboratories where the first night is associated with increased sleep latency, more wakefulness during the night, more poor-quality – Stage 1 sleep – and an increased delay to REM sleep.[15] However, the effect is not large and some studies have failed to find any first night effect on sleep quality at all.[16]

Environmental factors

Noise is a common cause of sleep disruption and complaint. There are marked variations between subjects in their sensitivity to awakening by noise,[17] and disturbability increases with age.[18] The cause and type of noise is also important; familiar unimportant noises may not waken an individual, but those of potential importance – for example the noise of a possible intruder – are effective at interrupting sleep. Crying babies may rapidly awaken mothers and the resulting sleep disturbance is a major cause of morbidity in many new mothers. Recurrent minor noises at levels too quiet to result in full awakening may produce sufficient sleep disruption to cause daytime sleepiness[19,20] without producing insomnia, as the subject is not aware of the interrupting episodes. Aircraft and road traffic noise may both markedly interfere with sleep pattern, although some habituation occurs. For some individuals living close to airports, major roads or railways, however, the noise may present a major and long-term threat to their quality of sleep. The use of earplugs and soundproofing can usually avoid the need to relocate, but sometimes that is the only acceptable solution. Long-term medication is not appropriate.

Too hot or too cold a bedroom will also interfere with sleep, producing more wakefulness through the night.[21] Personal comfort and habit may be important factors in determining optimal nocturnal temperature. Measures to produce a comfortable temperature in the room and bed usually suffice. Light intruding into the bedroom can interfere with sleep. Blackout blinds may be helpful, particularly in those who have to sleep by day.

An uncomfortable bed is often blamed for poor sleep quality. However, there is a lack of objective data indicating that bed type does consistently alter sleep quality. Familiarity and personal preference are important factors.

Caffeine

Sleep quality is impaired by caffeine,[22] although some are more sensitive to this effect than others. The sleep-disruptive effects of caffeine seem to be greater in the middle aged and elderly. A strong cup of coffee contains approximately 200 mg caffeine, and tea and cola drinks 50–75 mg. Effects may last up to 14 hours. Any patient with insomnia who takes more than 500 mg caffeine per day should try avoiding caffeine to see if this helps.

Alcohol

Consumption of alcohol in the evening may promote sleep onset but disturbs sleep later in the night, although this effect may decrease with regular alcohol use.[23]

Drugs

Insomnia can result either from a drug's direct effects or from drug withdrawal. Drugs causing insomnia include beta-blockers,[24,25] selective serotonin reuptake inhibitors (SSRIs),[26] theophyllines, according to some[27] but not all[28] studies, and other stimulant drugs such as amphetamines. Rebound insomnia is common following withdrawal from hypnotic or sedative drugs.[29] A detailed drug history should be sought in all patients with insomnia. In addition to prescribed medication, it is essential to ask about OTC medication use, including antihistamines, caffeine tablets and sympathomimetics, and also herbal medications, such as valerian root extract, cava-cava and chamomile, which are all sedatives, and ginseng which is a stimulant.

Shift work

Working alternating shift patterns, or a regular night shift but trying to maintain a nocturnal sleep pattern on days off, can be potent causes of both acute and chronic insomnia. As this is associated with circadian rhythm disorders it is discussed in Chapter 7. However, it is essential that anyone presenting with insomnia is asked about work patterns as well as sleep times.

CHRONIC INSOMNIA

When insomnia has persisted for at least six months it may be termed chronic. The classification of chronic insomnias is unsatisfactory with some systems sub-dividing and some lumping different types together. In the main, the latter approach will be adopted here with so-called primary and idiopathic chronic insomnias covered in this section.

In some patients, insomnia may have occurred all their lives and been present in childhood. This so-called primary insomnia is unusual and accounts for less than five per cent of cases of insomnia presenting to sleep clinics.[30] They may have an abnormality of neural control of the sleep–wake cycle, but the mechanism is not understood. It must be stressed that most children who sleep poorly will grow out of their problem with alteration in their life style; it is only the few who have persisting symptoms.

In many others, chronic insomnia is associated with a psychological element (Figure 6.1).[31] There is often learned sleep-preventing behaviour.[32] These patients with 'psychophysiological' insomnia constitute approximately 15 per cent of insomnia patients seen at sleep clinics.[30] They may have experienced a short-term stress which caused them to sleep poorly. They then feel tired and become increasingly anxious to get a good night's sleep and try hard to achieve this. When this secondary anxiety results in even greater difficulty sleeping, a vicious cycle is set up which is difficult to break. Such patients, who are trying 'too hard' to fall asleep in bed at night and failing, may paradoxically fall asleep readily in relaxed situations, such as watching television. These patients may also identify their own bedroom environment as non-conducive to sleep and may sleep better when away from home. All these features may persist even long after the original stress has passed. It is unclear whether persistence to chronic insomnia is more common in those with an underlying fragile sleep–wake control system, as has been suggested.[32]

Figure 6.1

Factors which may influence the development of chronic insomnia. (Adapted from Bearpark,[31] with permission.)

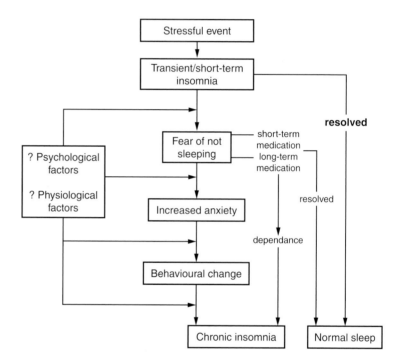

Diagnosis is based on the clinical features in the absence of underlying medical or psychiatric causes of insomnia. The features are excessive daily worries about inability to fall asleep in the absence of other major daytime anxieties. Sufferers show evidence of trying too hard to fall asleep in bed at night and paradoxical improvement in sleep quality when in a different environment. They may also exhibit increased agitation and muscle tension.

Some patients with chronic insomnia have been labelled as having 'sleep state misperception' in which the complaint of insomnia co-exists with EEG evidence of normal sleep duration and quality. Diagnostic difficulty is compounded by the following facts. Many subjects underestimate their sleep duration and sleep quality varies from night to night, so a single night's recording may have happened on a rare 'good' night. There is a wide range of normality of EEG-determined sleep duration and quality. Further, many such patients have a similar clinical picture to 'psychophysiological' insomnia. Despite repeated claims, there is no evidence that people are capable of going months or years without sleep and some such claimants may fall into the 'sleep state misperception' category.

Chronic insomnia can also be associated with a wide range of psychiatric disorders, which was the underlying cause in about a third of insomniacs presenting to a sleep clinic.[30] These include major depression, bipolar disorders, schizophrenia, anxiety disorders, personality disorders and dementia.

There are a large number of medical causes of insomnia. Many are covered elsewhere in this book, some – such as illnesses causing chronic pain – are self-evident, but some require specific coverage.

In **chronic renal failure**, insomnia is common. This is sometimes associated with PLMD or OSAHS.[33]

Chronic fatigue syndrome (ME, 'myalgic encephalopathy') is often associated with insomnia and increased daytime sleepiness. As there is no diagnostic test for this condition, it is important to ensure that an adequate sleep history has been taken and that a primary sleep disorder such as OSAHS has not been missed.

Fibromyalgia is characterized by chronic myalgias with point tenderness in specified locations.[34] Many complain of insomnia and chronic fatigue. Success has been reported with exercise programmes, tricyclic antidepressants, chlorpromazine and cyclobenzaprine.

Tourette's syndrome is a complex of multiple tics, associated with grunting, snorting and sniffing and the involuntary utterance of profanities. No neurological cause has been identified and there is no familial tendency. Approximately 50 per cent of sufferers report insomnia and there is also an increase in sleep walking. Haloperidol, clonazepam and clonidine have been reported to be effective.

INSOMNIA IN THE ELDERLY

Nearly 60 per cent of older adults complain of sleeping difficulties.[35,36] Around 30 per cent of those over the age of 65 report difficulty maintaining sleep, whereas 20 per cent report difficulty falling asleep and a similar number report early morning wakening.[36] About 40 per cent of prescriptions for hypnotics are to over 60-year-olds.[37]

Overall sleep requirements fall with increasing age, according to many[38,39] but not all[40] studies. One of the factors contributing to this basic confusion includes the question of whether total sleep time over a 24-hour period decreases in the elderly. There is general agreement that nocturnal sleep times fall but this is probably because older people have greater opportunities for daytime napping than those in employment or looking after children.

The elderly certainly have an increased frequency of nocturnal wakenings, especially late in the night.[41–43] There is evidence they waken more readily in response to noise[44] and have greater difficulty in getting back to sleep once woken.[45] Other differences in sleep include shorter stages 3/4 sleep due to a decline in the amplitude of slow waves and a slight decrease in the amount of REM sleep.[46]

The combination of increased nocturnal wakening, difficulty in falling asleep again and decreased nocturnal sleep duration are presumably major factors in the relatively high prevalence of the complaint of insomnia in the elderly. Other factors favouring sleep difficulties include the decreased exercise taken by older less physically well people, less exposure to bright light to synchronize circadian and sleep–wake rhythms, and lower levels of circulating melatonin in the elderly.[47]

Pain due to osteoarthritis or other illness may also contribute to their insomnia. Heart and respiratory disease are also statistically associated with insomnia.[48]

Assessment of patients with insomnia

As with most areas of medicine, one starts with a full history and physical examination. The history is the most important element in diagnosis[49,50] and should concentrate on the perceived problems with sleep, ability to initiate and maintain sleep, bedtime, final wakening time and daytime sequelae. The duration and precipitants of wakenings should be clarified as well as what steps patients have taken to try to remedy the situation. Daytime activity, naps, caffeine, alcohol and drug ingestion and work routines must be documented. Depression, anxiety, other psychological problems and heightened arousal should be sought.[49] The co-existence of other sleep-related disorders should be considered, especially OSAHS and periodic limb movements during sleep. Most sleep centres find that sleep questionnaires for patients and their bed partner are the best way to gather this material initially. Gathering information from the partner independently can be very useful, especially when sleep state misperception is a possibility. Responses will need to be clarified by direct questioning. Physical examination is often normal, but evidence of medical conditions which might contribute to insomnia – such as arthritis or sleep apnoea – should be sought. Psychological and/or psychiatric assessments may need to be performed in some patients.

The first level of investigation is often to have patients complete a sleep diary for a few weeks. There are numerous diaries available on paper or on the internet (for example, http://www.sleepfoundation.org/publications/diary.html) but a simple one is shown in Table 6.1.

Sleep diary for: ....

Please shade the boxes to show when you slept each day and night.
For example, if you slept from 2 pm until 4 pm and then again from midnight until 4 am, the record would look like this:

Noon	2	4	6	8	10	12	2	4	6	8	10	12

Total hours slept: 6

Please list all of your medications below (include herbal and over the counter (OTC) medications that you take):
....
....

Please add any notes that you feel are important to know about your sleep:
....
....

Dates: /   /   /   until   /   /   /

Monday

		Daytime					Night-time					
12	2	4	6	8	10	12mn	2	4	6	8	10	Noon

Hours slept:

Tuesday

		Daytime					Night-time					
12	2	4	6	8	10	12mn	2	4	6	8	10	Noon

Hours slept:

Wednesday

		Daytime					Night-time					
12	2	4	6	8	10	12mn	2	4	6	8	10	Noon

Hours slept:

Thursday

		Daytime					Night-time					
12	2	4	6	8	10	12mn	2	4	6	8	10	Noon

Hours slept:

Friday

		Daytime					Night-time					
12	2	4	6	8	10	12mn	2	4	6	8	10	Noon

Hours slept:

Saturday

		Daytime					Night-time					
12	2	4	6	8	10	12mn	2	4	6	8	10	Noon

Hours slept:

Sunday

		Daytime					Night-time					
12	2	4	6	8	10	12mn	2	4	6	8	10	Noon

Hours slept:

Table 6.1
Example of a sleep diary

More complex diaries may be helpful in certain situations with specific questions addressing:

- When the problem began.
- Bedtime and rise time.
- Time to fall asleep.
- Number of nocturnal wakenings.
- Total sleep duration.
- Daytime naps.
- Shift schedules (where relevant).
- Number of caffeinated drinks.
- Alcohol consumption.
- Mood.
- Psychiatric or medical disorders.
- Medication.
- Creeping/crawling/uncomfortable feelings in legs relieved by moving them (suggests restless leg syndrome).
- Partner reports repeated leg jerks during sleep (PLMD) or loud snoring/apnoeas (sleep apnoea/hypopnoea).
- Comments.

This is usually sufficient investigation and rarely is it necessary in insomnia to move to the next level of investigation in order to add some objectivity by estimating sleep times. This can be done using portable movement detectors, usually combined with the simultaneous completion of a diary. Such actigraphy devices usually are worn like wrist watches and give fair estimates of sleep duration from periods of immobility.[51,52] The results may be useful both in terms of demonstrating to patients and their relatives that they are sleeping for longer than they think, and to monitor improvements with therapy. They are also useful to document and monitor treatment in sleep phase disorders (*see* Chapter 7).

The role of polysomnography in insomnia is debated. In most patients polysomnography has little role, and none if there is an identifiable cause for insomnia or if the problem is sleep onset insomnia, psychophysiological insomnia or phase alteration. If, however, the problem is isolated sleep maintenance insomnia then polysomnography may identify OSAHS or periodic limb movements, but such investigation should be guided by a detailed history from both the patient and the sleep partner.

Treatment of insomnia

The management of a patient's insomnia must be tailored to the individual's needs. In the case of short-term insomnia, the steps are often self-evident, as discussed above. This section will focus on the treatment of long-term insomnia, which is often challenging. The goal should be to achieve better sleep and patients must be asked to realize from an early stage that perfect sleep is not always achievable.

Management consists of several elements. The general advice on sleeping habits is applicable to all patients with chronic insomnia, the applicability of other elements will vary.

GENERAL ADVICE

Patients should be asked to follow some simple rules (*see* Table 6.2):

1 **Don't have a fixed bedtime**. Go to bed and lie down when you are sleepy, not because it is time for bed.
2 **Do have a fixed get up time**. Getting up at a set time allows the circadian rhythms to be firmly established and avoids the phase delay syndrome developing. Do not try to sleep longer because you felt you had a bad night.
3 **Do limit your activities in bed**. Bed should be a place to sleep, not one to lie watching television or reading. Work should not be done in the bedroom. As sexual intercourse is followed by sleepiness for many, this may be permitted, or even encouraged.
4 **Do not stay in bed if fully awake**. After failing to fall asleep in about 20 minutes, or a similar duration of full awakening through the night, patients should get up, go to another room and do something relaxing in subdued lighting. Once the next wave of sleepiness comes along, go back to bed and catch it.
5 **Do not nap during the day**. This not only decreases sleepiness at bedtime but also confuses the circadian clock.
6 **Do exercise**. Fit people sleep better, and exercise during the day should be encouraged. However, vigorous exercise within two to three hours of bedtime can delay sleep onset.
7 **Do have a bedtime ritual**. Different patterns work for different people. Some benefit from a light snack, a hot milky drink or listening to relaxing music. Large amounts of food or alcohol and caffeine-containing drinks should be avoided. Smoking near bedtime or during wakenings should be avoided as nicotine is a stimulant.
8 **Do banish clocks**. Watching the time going past is not only a depressing night-time activity for many insomniacs, it can generate considerable anxiety. Furthermore, some may wake themselves fully to read the clock and then fail to get back to sleep. Clocks should either be banned from the bedroom or turned face away from the bed if an alarm is needed. This

means that the 20 minutes of wakefulness which leads to leaving the bedroom (point 4) must be an estimate, NOT a measured time.

9 **Do not use bed as a place to solve problems.** Some people only find time to think about their current anxieties when lying in bed at night. If this is a feature of patients' insomnia, they should be advised to set aside a defined block of 'worry time' before going to bed.

10 **Do not worry if you do not sleep.** Although this is much easier said than done, patients should be educated about the wide differences in sleep requirements and that one can function well on less than perfect sleep quality and duration.

Table 6.2

How to improve your sleep

> Don't have a fixed bedtime
> Do have a fixed get up time
> Do limit your activities in bed
> Do not stay in bed if fully awake
> Do not nap during the day
> Do exercise
> Do have a bedtime ritual
> Do banish clocks
> Do not use bed as a place to solve problems
> Do not worry if you do not sleep

Some of these pieces of advice, especially rules 1, 3, 4 and 9, are designed to imprint the concept that bed is for sleep only and have been termed 'stimulus control therapy'.[53] Others are general measures to facilitate good sleep and may be called 'sleep hygiene'. Patients should be encouraged to follow these instructions strictly for several weeks in order to establish a new sleep rhythm. Reinforcement may be needed and the input of nurses trained in sleep medicine can be very helpful. Patients may be helped by further information from books[54,55] or the internet, such as the British Sleep Foundation (www.britishsleepfoundation.org.uk), National Sleep Foundation (www.sleepfoundation.org) or Sleep Home Pages (www.sleephomepages.org).

These instructions will often suffice on their own but when they do not, a careful enquiry should be made into the reasons for failure and, specifically, which pieces of advice are not being followed and why. For example, patients may not wait until they are sleepy to go to bed because they wish to have the same bedtime as their partner. Sometimes discussion with both parties may produce the understanding required to reach a satisfactory solution. Others may object to some of the rules, citing the examples of friends or family members who always read or watch TV in bed and sleep well. They should be helped to understand that such behaviour is fine for good sleepers, but not for poor ones.

Some patients worry excessively about sleep loss, have unrealistic expectations about sleep requirements and may attribute many of their other life problems inappropriately to their insomnia. In them, cognitive behavioural therapy (CBT) may be helpful. This first identifies the patient's misperceptions about sleep, often by use of a questionnaire.[56] Cognitive therapy is aimed at changing insomniacs' views of the sleep problem from one in which they are victims of a sleep disorder to one in which they are capable of coping with the problem. Attempts are made to explain to patients that they can control many of the determinants of their own sleep quality. Another goal is to address some of the misattributions of the consequences of insomnia; few of their daytime symptoms are likely to be due to their perceived poor sleep. Many have unrealistic expectations of sleep duration which need rectified. For example, those who believe that eight hours' sleep is needed to function normally should be asked to question their own experience and see if this has been the case. Finally, cognitive therapy should be directed to educate patients that it is not insomnia that is upsetting their life and that they can cope and perform well even in the presence of insomnia. In this way cognitive therapy allays the hyperarousal associated with insomnia which tends to perpetuate the problem. CBT may be led by physicians, psychologists or nurses trained in these techniques.[57]

Patients with psychophysiological insomnia may have a major problem with tension at bedtime getting them into a vicious circle, in which previous poor sleep leads to anxiety and anticipation of poor sleep, which becomes a self-fulfilling prophecy. This can be often be helped by developing relaxation skills.[58] None of the many relaxation techniques have been shown to be better than the others. A wind-down time prior to sleep should be instituted during the second half of the evening and an absolute bar placed on work or exercise in the hour and a half before bedtime. After getting into bed, a relaxation routine should be practised, such as concentrating on breathing deeply and slowly in time to a thought – but not vocalized – 'in, out', relaxing major muscle groups in sequence, including the arms, face, neck, shoulders, stomach, back and legs. These exercises should be repeated during major awakenings during the night. It is often helpful to develop them as a skill to be used also during the day to aid relaxation. Some find audiotapes of relaxing exercises or music before bed useful.

Sleep restriction: sleep restriction can be an effective treatment in patients with insomnia.[59] This strategy matches patients' permitted time in bed to their total estimated sleep time. For example, if the patient must get up for work each day at 7 am and estimates that his or her total sleep duration is five hours, he or she would be asked to delay bedtime until 2 am. Sleep restriction is based on the observation that insomniacs have low sleep efficiency,[59] and the concern that additional time spent awake in bed may increase arousal.

Insomnia in the elderly

The management of insomnia in the elderly is broadly similar to that in younger patient, but some additional points are relevant. First, it is particularly important to try to prevent daytime and evening naps in this population in order to consolidate night-time sleep. Second, gentle exercise in the daytime should be encouraged,[60] this serving the dual function of promoting sleep directly as well as preventing napping while exercise is being taken. Third, they should try to get daily exposure to daylight to synchronize their circadian clocks. This is particularly a problem in the institutionalized old. Fourth, nocturnal sleep requirements may fall with age – although this is debatable (*see* page 155) – and patients should be reassured that less nocturnal sleep and more nocturnal wakenings are common. Thus expectations may need to be adjusted. Further, the other therapies offered for chronic insomnia may also be helpful in the elderly, especially CBT.[61]

Late evening bright light therapy may improve both sleep and daytime performance in the elderly patient with sleep maintenance insomnia in comparison to sham therapy.[62,63] The precise role for light therapy requires further study but this is a promising potential non-pharmacological approach. On the other hand, placebo-controlled trials in the elderly have shown no benefit from melatonin therapy given before sleep, as sustained release at bedtime or when taken later in the sleep period.[64]

HYPNOTIC THERAPY

Although all sleep physicians agree that hypnotic drugs should rarely be used in insomnia, with stances varying from never to occasionally, the fact is that hypnotic agents are still very widely prescribed.[65,66] In addition, many, perhaps 40 per cent of insomniacs,[3] use OTC medications, such as antihistamines or alcohol, to try to help them sleep.

Hypnotic agents have a role in some cases of acute insomnia where there is a clear stressor disrupting sleep, such as bereavement, or attempting to sleep on planes or trains. Nevertheless, all other reasonable non-pharmacological steps should be tried first – such as simple measures like earplugs, bedtime routines and relaxation therapy. The use of hypnotic agents should be kept to the smallest number of nights possible and certainly to less than two weeks in all situations.

The role of hypnotics in chronic insomnia is much more controversial. The counsel of perfection held by most sleep physicians is that there is no role, but in practice two-thirds of prescriptions for hypnotic agents go to chronic users.[66] There is no evidence of improvement compared to placebo in either subjective or objective sleep quality in chronic insomniacs after five weeks' therapy with triazolam, flurazepam[67] or zolpidem.[68] In addition, daytime cognitive function is impaired with use of hypnotic agents, more markedly by long-acting but also by short-acting hypnotics.[69,70] There is also evidence that long-term nightly use of hypnotic agents has a similar effect on mortality to smoking at least 20 cigarettes per day.[71] Thus, patients often take hypnotic agents in the hope of improving daytime performance when in fact they impair daytime function, do not improve sleep and may increase mortality. Hypnotic agents should not be used long term.

Some advocate the use of hypnotics in conjunction with other approaches when therapy for chronic insomnia is initiated.[4,72] Such use should not be for more than four weeks, but the problem then is stopping the drugs as there is rebound deterioration in sleep on withdrawal from the drug.[29,73] Rebound deterioration can occur after even as little as one night of therapy with a hypnotic agent,[74] but is commoner when larger hypnotic dosages have been used.[75] The rebound deterioration after withdrawal often reinforces patients' belief that they cannot sleep well without the drug. Tapering off the drug dosage over many days decreases rebound insomnia,[73] and this is the best way to try to get patients off the drugs, in conjunction with providing support and non-pharmacological treatment.

The choice of hypnotic therapy should include consideration of half-life, therapeutic index and drug dosage. The biological half-life of hypnotics varies widely (Table 6.3). Unless daytime sedation or late in the night hypnotic effects are being actively sought, shorter half-life drugs are preferable.

Benzodiazepines and the newer non-benzodiazepines which act selectively on some benzodiazepine receptors – zolpidem, zaleplon and zopiclone – are relatively safe in overdose and have good therapeutic ratios. The newer

Table 6.3
Hypnotic drugs

Half-life (hours)	Drug	Dose (mg)
Less than 4 hours	Trizolam	0.125–0.25
	Zolpidem	5–10 (–20 if patient less than 65 years old)
	Zaleplon	5 (–10 if patient less than 65 years old)
4–8 hours	Zopiclone	3.75 (–7.5 if patient less than 65 years old)
	Temezepam	15–30
	Lorazepam	0.5–2
More than 8 hours	Lormetrazepam	1–2
	Nitrazepam	5–10
	Clonazepam	0.5–2
	Diazepam	2–10
	Flurazepam	15–30

receptor drugs seem to be broadly similar to the benzodiazepines in their effects on sleep, daytime function[76] and potential dependence[77] and these drugs do not have sufficient advantages to make them the drugs of exclusive choice at present.

Hypnotic drug dosage should be kept to the minimum that is effective. Daytime side-effects are frequently the result of using too high a dose in an effort to achieve efficacy. Care must be taken not to do this. As hypnotic agents are frequently used in the elderly in whom drug metabolism is usually slowed, lower dosages of shorter-acting drugs should be used in the old wherever possible.

Small doses of antidepressant medication may be used to facilitate sleep instead of conventional hypnotic agents. Some of these medications (for example, trazodone, nefazodone) have the theoretical advantage of reduced REM sleep and slow wave sleep suppression.[78,79] However, some antidepressant medications may exacerbate periodic leg movements during sleep.[80] Caution should be used when treating elderly insomniacs with these agents because of an increased risk of falls due to drowsiness and postural hypotension.

Useful reviews

- Kripke, D.E. (2000) Chronic hypnotic use: deadly risks, doubtful benefit. *Sleep Medicine Reviews*, **4**, 5–20.
- National Centre on Sleep Disorders Research Insomnia Working Group. (1999) Insomnia: assessment and management in primary care. *Sleep*, **22**, S402–S408.
- Sateia, M.J., Doghramji, K., Hauri, P.J., Morin, C.M. (2000) Evaluation of chronic insomnia. An American Academy of Sleep Medicine review. *Sleep*, **23**, 243–308.
- Morin, C.M., Hauri, P.J., Espie, C.A., Spielman, A.J., Buysse, D.J., Bootzin, R.R. (1999) Nonpharmacologic treatment of chronic insomnia. An American Academy of Sleep Medicine review. *Sleep*, **22**, 1134–56.

References

1   Mellinger, G.D., Balter, M.B., Uhlenhuth, E.H. (1985) Insomnia and its treatment. Prevalence and correlates. *Arch. Gen. Psychiatry*, **42**, 225–32.

2   Ford, D.E., Kamerow, D.B. (1989) Epidemiologic study of sleep disturbances and psychiatric disorders. An opportunity for prevention? *JAMA*, **262**, 1479–84.

3   National Sleep Foundation. (1991) *Sleep in America: A National Survey of US Adults*. Princeton, NJ: Gallup Organization. (Ref Type: Pamphlet)

4   Costa, eS.J., Chase, M., Sartorius, N., Roth, T. (1996) Special report from a symposium held by the World Health Organization and the World Federation of Sleep Research Societies: an overview of insomnias and related disorders – recognition, epidemiology, and rational management. *Sleep*, **19**, 412–16.

5   Walsh, J.K., Engelhardt, C.L. (1999) The direct economic costs of insomnia in the United States for 1995. *Sleep*, **22** (Suppl. 2), S386–S393.

6   Leger, D., Levy, E., Paillard, M. (1999) The direct costs of insomnia in France. *Sleep*, **22** (Suppl. 2), S394–S401.

7   Mendelson, W.B., Garnett, D., Gillin, J.C., Weingartner, H. (1984) The experience of insomnia and daytime and nighttime functioning. *Psychiatry Res.*, **12**, 235–50.

8   Seidel, W.F., Ball, S., Cohen, S., Patterson, N., Yost, D., Dement, W.C. (1984) Daytime alertness in relation to mood, performance, and nocturnal sleep in chronic insomniacs and noncomplaining sleepers. *Sleep*, 7, 230–8.

9   Mendelson, W.B., James, S.P., Garnett, D., Sack, D.A., Rosenthal, N.E. (1986) A psychophysiological study of insomnia. *Psychiatry Res.*, **19**, 267–84.

10 Stepanski, E., Zorick, F., Roehrs, T., Young, D., Roth, T. (1988) Daytime alertness in patients with chronic insomnia compared with asymptomatic control subjects. *Sleep*, **11**, 54–60.

11 Riedel, B.W., Lichstein, K.L. (2000) Insomnia and daytime functioning. *Sleep Medicine Reviews*, **4**, 277–98.

12 National Commission on Sleep Disorders Research. (1993) *Wake up America: A National Sleep Alert*. Washington: US Government Printing Office.

13 Cernovsky, Z.Z. (1984) Life stress measures and reported frequency of sleep disorders. *Percept. Mot. Skills*, **58**, 39–49.

14 Torsvall, L., Akerstedt, T. (1988) Disturbed sleep while being on-call: an EEG study of ships' engineers. *Sleep*, **11**, 35–8.

15 Agnew, H.W., Webb, W.B., Williams. R.L. (1966) The first night effect: an EEG study of sleep. *Psychophysiology*, **2**, 263–6.

16 Kader, G.A., Griffin, P.T. (1983) Reevaluation of the phenomena of the first night effect. *Sleep*, **6**, 67–71.

17 Rechtschaffen, A., Hauri, P., Zeitlin, M. (1966) Auditory awakening

thresholds in REM and NREM sleep stages. *Percept. Mot. Skills*, **22**, 927–42.

18   Roth, T., Kramer, M., Trinder, J. (1972) The effect of noise during sleep on the sleep patterns of different age groups. *Can. Psychiatr. Assoc. J.*, **17** (Suppl. 2), SS197.

19   Roehrs, T., Merlotti, L., Petrucelli, N., Stepanski, E., Roth, T. (1994) Experimental sleep fragmentation. *Sleep*, **17**, 438–43.

20   Martin, S.E., Engleman, H.M., Deary, I.J., Douglas, N.J. (1996) The effect of sleep fragmentation on daytime function. *Am. J. Respir. Crit. Care Med.*, **153**, 1328–32.

21   Haskell, E.H., Palca, J.W., Walker, J.M., Berger, R.J., Heller, H.C. (1981) The effects of high and low ambient temperatures on human sleep stages. *Electroencephalogr. Clin. Neurophysiol.*, **51**, 494–501.

22   Rosenthal, L., Roehrs, T., Zwyghuizen-Doorenbos, A., Plath, D., Roth, T. (1991) Alerting effects of caffeine after normal and restricted sleep. *Neuropsychopharmacology*, **4**, 103–8.

23   Rundell, O.H., Lester, B.K., Griffiths, W.J., Williams, H.L. (1972) Alcohol and sleep in young adults. *Psychopharmacologia*, **26**, 201–18.

24   Kostis, J.B., Rosen, R.C. (1987) Central nervous system effects of beta-adrenergic-blocking drugs: the role of ancillary properties. *Circulation*, **75**, 204–12.

25   Kostis, J.B., Rosen, R.C., Holzer, B.C., Randolph, C., Taska, L.S., Miller, M.H. (1990) CNS side effects of centrally-active antihypertensive agents: a prospective, placebo-controlled study of sleep, mood state, and cognitive and sexual function in hypertensive males. *Psychopharmacology*, **102**, 163–70.

26   Grimsley, S.R., Jann, M.W. (1992) Paroxetine, sertraline, and fluvoxamine: new selective serotonin reuptake inhibitors. *Clin. Pharm.*, **11**, 930–57.

27   Rhind, G.B., Connaughton, J.J., McFie, J., Douglas, N.J., Flenley, D.C. (1985) Sustained release choline theophyllinate in nocturnal asthma. *BMJ*, **291**, 1605–7.

28   Fitzpatrick, M.F., Engleman, H.M., Boellert, F., McHardy, R., Shapiro, C.M., Deary, I.J. *et al.* (1992) Effect of therapeutic theophylline levels on the sleep quality and daytime cognitive performance of normal subjects. *Am. Rev. Respir. Dis.*, **145**, 1355–8.

29   Roehrs, T., Vogel, G., Roth, T. (1990) Rebound insomnia: its determinants and significance. *Am. J. Med.*, **88**, 39S–42S.

30   Coleman, R.M., Roffwarg, H.P., Kennedy, S.J., Guilleminault, C., Cinque, J., Cohn, M.A. *et al.* (1982) Sleep–wake disorders based on a polysomnographic diagnosis. A national cooperative study. *JAMA*, **247**, 997–1003.

31 Bearpark, H. (1994) Insomnia: causes, effects and treatment, in R. Cooper (ed). *Sleep*, pp. 587–613. London: Chapman & Hall.

32 Hauri, P., Fisher, J. (1986) Persistent psychophysiologic (learned) insomnia. *Sleep*, **9**, 38–53.

33 Hallett, M., Burden, S., Stewart, D., Mahony, J., Farrell, P. (1995) Sleep apnea in end-stage renal disease patients on hemodialysis and continuous ambulatory peritoneal dialysis. *ASAIO J*, **41**, M435–M441.

34 C-ote, K.A., Moldofsky, H. (1997) Sleep, daytime symptoms, and cognitive performance in patients with fibromyalgia. *J. Rheumatol.*, **24**, 2014–23.

35 Bliwise, D.L. (1993) Sleep in normal aging and dementia. *Sleep*, **16**, 40–81.

36 Foley, D.J., Monjan, A.A., Brown, S.L., Simonsick, E.M., Wallace, R.B., Blazer, D.G. (1995) Sleep complaints among elderly persons: an epidemiologic study of three communities. *Sleep*, **18**, 425–32.

37 Kripke, D.F., Simons, R.N., Garfinkel, L., Hammond, E.C. (1979) Short and long sleep and sleeping pills. Is increased mortality associated? *Arch. Gen. Psychiatry*, **36**, 103–16.

38 Gillin, J.C., Duncan, W.C., Murphy, D.L., Post, R.M., Wehr, T.A., Goodwin, F.K. *et al.* (1981) Age-related changes in sleep in depressed and normal subjects. *Psychiatry Res.*, **4**, 73–8.

39 Bixler, E.O., Kales, A., Jacoby, J.A., Soldatos, C.R., Vela-Bueno, A. (1984) Nocturnal sleep and wakefulness: effects of age and sex in normal sleepers. *Int. J. Neurosci.*, **23**, 33–42.

40 Tune, G.S. (1969 The influence of age and temperament on the adult human sleep–wakefulness pattern. *Br. J. Psychol.*, **60**, 431–41.

41 Reynolds, C.F., Kupfer, D.J., Taska, L.S., Hoch, C.C., Spiker, D.G., Sewitch, D.E. *et al.* (1985) EEG sleep in elderly depressed, demented, and healthy subjects. *Biol. Psychiatry*, **20**, 431–42.

42 Hirshkowitz, M., Moore, C.A., Hamilton, C.R. III, Rando, K.C., Karacan, I. (1992) Polysomnography of adults and elderly: sleep architecture, respiration, and leg movement. *J. Clin. Neurophysiol.*, **9**, 56–62.

43 Mathur, R., Douglas, N.J. (1995) Frequency of EEG arousals from nocturnal sleep in normal subjects. *Sleep*, **18**, 330–3.

44 Zepelin, H., McDonald, C.S., Zammit, G.K. (1984) Effects of age on auditory awakening thresholds. *J. Gerontol.*, **39**, 294–300.

45 Webb, W., Campbell, S. (1980) Duration of non-laboratory sleep in an aging population. *Sleep Res.*, **9**, 128.

46 Benca, R.M., Obermeyer, W.H., Thisted, R.A., Gillin, J.C. (1992) Sleep and psychiatric disorders. A meta-analysis. *Arch. Gen. Psychiatry*, **49**, 651–68.

47 Sack, R.L., Lewy, A.J., Erb, D.L., Vollmer, W.M., Singer, C.M. (1986) Human melatonin production decreases with age. *J. Pineal Res.*, **3**, 379–88.

48 Foley, D.J., Monjan, A., Simonsick, E.M., Wallace, R.B., Blazer, D.G. (1999) Incidence and remission of insomnia among elderly adults: an epidemiologic study of 6800 persons over three years. *Sleep*, **22** (Suppl. 2), S366–S372.

49 Chesson, A., Hartse, K., Anderson, W.M., Davila, D., Johnson, S., Littner, M. *et al.* (2000) Practice parameters for the evaluation of chronic insomnia. An American Academy of Sleep Medicine report. Standards of Practice Committee of the American Academy of Sleep Medicine. *Sleep*, **23**, 237–41.

50 Sateia, M.J., Doghramji, K., Hauri, P.J., Morin, C.M. (2000) Evaluation of chronic insomnia. An American Academy of Sleep Medicine review. *Sleep*, **23**, 243–308.

51 Cole, R.J., Kripke, D.F., Gruen, W., Mullaney, D.J., Gillin, J.C. (1992) Automatic sleep/wake identification from wrist activity. *Sleep*, **15**, 461–9.

52 Sadeh, A., Alster, J., Urbach, D., Lavie, P. (1989) Actigraphically based automatic bedtime sleep-wake scoring: validity and clinical applications. *Journal of Ambulatory Monitoring*, **2**, 209–16.

53 Morin, C.M., Hauri, P.J., Espie, C.A., Spielman, A.J., Buysse, D.J., Bootzin, R.R. (1999) Nonpharmacologic treatment of chronic insomnia. An American Academy of Sleep Medicine review. *Sleep*, **22**, 1134–56.

54 Bearpark, H. (1994) *Overcoming Insomnia*. Woollahra, NSW, Australia: Gore & Osment.

55 Hauri, P., Linde, S. (1996) *No More Sleepless Nights: A Proven Program to Conquer Insomnia*. New York: Wiley.

56 Sloan, E.P., Hauri, P., Bootzin, R., Morin, C., Stevenson, M., Shapiro, C.M. (1993) The nuts and bolts of behavioral therapy for insomnia. *J. Psychosom. Res.*, **37** (Suppl. 1), 19–37.

57 Espie, C.A., Inglis, S.J., Tessier, S., Harvey, L. (2001) The clinical effectiveness of cognitive behaviour therapy for chronic insomnia: implementation and evaluation of a sleep clinic in general medical practice. *Behav. Res. Ther.*, **39**, 45–60.

58 Espie, C.A. (1993) ABC of sleep disorders. Practical management of insomnia: behavioural and cognitive techniques. *BMJ*, **306**, 509–11.

59 Spielman, A.J., Saskin, P., Thorpy, M.J. (1987) Treatment of chronic insomnia by restriction of time in bed. *Sleep*, **10**, 45–56.

60 King, A.C., Oman, R.F., Brassington, G.S., Bliwise, D.L., Haskell, W.L. (1997) Moderate-intensity exercise and self-rated quality of sleep in older adults. A randomized controlled trial. *JAMA*, **277**, 32–7.

61 Morin, C.M., Colecchi, C., Stone, J., Sood, R., Brink, D. (1999) Behavioral and pharmacological therapies for late-life insomnia: a randomized controlled trial. *JAMA*, **281**, 991–9.

62 Campbell, S.S., Dawson, D., Anderson, M.W. (1993) Alleviation of sleep maintenance insomnia with timed exposure to bright light. *J. Am. Geriatr. Soc.*, **41**, 829–36.

63 Murphy, P.J., Campbell, S.S. (1996) Enhanced performance in elderly subjects following bright light treatment of sleep maintenance insomnia. *J. Sleep. Res.*, **5**, 165–72.

64 Hughes, R.J., Sack, R.L., Lewy, A.J. (1998) The role of melatonin and circadian phase in age-related sleep- maintenance insomnia: assessment in a clinical trial of melatonin replacement. *Sleep*, **21**, 52–68.

65 Ashton, H., Golding, J.F. (1989) Tranquillisers: prevalence, predictors and possible consequences. Data from a large United Kingdom survey. *Br. J. Addict.*, **84**, 541–6.

66 Kripke, D.F. (2000) Chronic hypnotic use:deadly risks, doubtful benefit. *Sleep Medicine Reviews*, **4**, 5–20.

67 Mitler, M.M., Seidel, W.F., Van den, H.J., Greenblatt, D.J., Dement, W.C. (1984) Comparative hypnotic effects of flurazepam, triazolam, and placebo: a long-term simultaneous nighttime and daytime study. *J. Clin. Psychopharmacol.*, **4**, 2–13.

68 Scharf, M.B., Roth, T., Vogel, G.W., Walsh, J.K. (1994) A multicenter, placebo-controlled study evaluating zolpidem in the treatment of chronic insomnia. *J. Clin. Psychiatry*, **55**, 192–9.

69 Morgan, K. (1994) Hypnotic drugs, psychomotor performance and ageing. *J. Sleep Res.*, **3**, 1–15.

70 Woods, J.H., Katz, J.L., Winger, G. (1992) Benzodiazepines: use, abuse, and consequences. *Pharmacol. Rev.*, **44**, 151–347.

71 Kripke, D.F., Klauber, M.R., Wingard, D.L., Fell, R.L., Assmus, J.D., Garfinkel, L. (1998) Mortality hazard associated with prescription hypnotics. *Biol. Psychiatry*, **43**, 687–93.

72 Roth, T. (1996) Management of insomniac patients. *Sleep*, **19**, S52–S53.

73 Roehrs, T., Merlotti, L., Zorick, F., Roth, T. (1992) Rebound insomnia in normals and patients with insomnia after abrupt and tapered discontinuation. *Psychopharmacology*, **1992**, 108, 67–71.

74 Merlotti, L., Roehrs, T., Zorick, F., Roth, T. (1991) Rebound insomnia: duration of use and individual differences. *J. Clin. Psychopharmacol.*, **11**, 368–73.

75 Roehrs, T.A., Zorick, F.J., Wittig, R.M., Roth, T. (1986) Dose determinants of rebound insomnia. *Br. J. Clin. Pharmacol.*, **22**, 143–7.

76 Rush, C.R. (1998) Behavioral pharmacology of zolpidem relative to benzodiazepines: a review. *Pharmacol. Biochem. Behav.*, **61**, 253–69.

77 Heydorn, W.E. (2000) Zaleplon – a review of a novel sedative hypnotic used in the treatment of insomnia. *Expert. Opin. Investig. Drugs*, **9**, 841–58.

78 Thase, M.E. (2000) Treatment issues related to sleep and depression. *J. Clin. Psychiatry*, **61** (Suppl. 11), 46–50.

79 DeVane, C.L. (1998) Differential pharmacology of newer antidepressants. *J. Clin. Psychiatry*, **59** (Suppl. 20), 85–93.

80 Coleman, R.M., Pollak, C.P., Weitzman, E.D. (1980) Periodic movements in sleep (nocturnal myoclonus): relation to sleep disorders. *Ann. Neurol.*, **8**, 416–21.

Circadian rhythm disorders

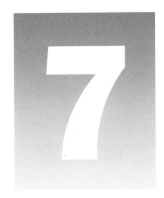

Introduction to circadian rhythms

Many body functions are under circadian control, including hormone secretion, body temperature, cellular and enzymatic function and sleep. The circadian clock is situated in the supra-chiasmatic nucleus, in the anterior hypothalamus immediately above the optic chiasm.

LIGHT

Light is the principle synchronizer of this central circadian pacemaker and this input comes via the retino-hypothalamic tract.[1] Exposure to light during a time when it is usually dark will alter circadian rhythms. It used to be thought that only very bright light equivalent to daylight could effect the circadian pacemaker but recent studies show that even ordinary room lighting can have a lesser but still significant effect on this pacemaker[2] (Figure 7.1). The magnitude of the phase shifting effect is proportional to the cube root of the light intensity.[3] Light exposure immediately before or soon after dark onset delays the circadian clock while light towards the end of darkness or early in the daylight period advances circadian rhythms.

Light is by far the most important circadian phase setting influence in man. The only other factor convincingly shown to change circadian phase is exercise, night-time exercise delaying the circadian clock.[4]

MELATONIN

Melatonin is secreted from the pineal gland during the hours of darkness, thus blood levels are usually high at night and low by day. Exposure to light produces a rapid decrease in circulating levels. The suprachiasmatic nucleus has a high concentration of melatonin receptors and there is some evidence that melatonin administered in physiological doses can phase shift the circadian clock.[5] Melatonin administration before the body's normal peak

Figure 7.1
Dose-response curve of light intensity on phase shift. Each light intensity was given for five hours per day for eight days. (From Boivirt,[2] with permission.)

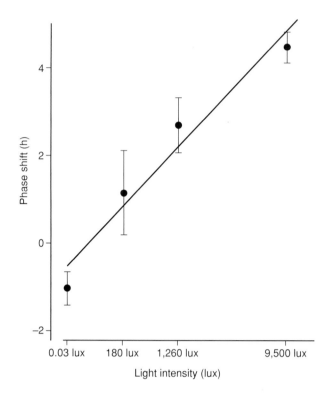

advances the sleep–wake cycle, whereas later administration – in the morning – delays the cycle. Melatonin has a direct hypnotic effect leading to shorter sleep onset in some, but not all, studies.[6] The side-effects of melatonin use include coronary and pulmonary artery constriction, but their long-term significance is unclear.

Shift work

The sleep disturbance caused by shift work has only recently been recognized as a major cause of morbidity in the community. Problems are most common in those on rotating shifts, for example some work 4 am to noon one week, noon to 8 pm the next week and 8 pm to 4 am the next. Workers on permanent night shift who revert to nocturnal sleep patterns on their nights off are also prone to sleep disturbance. This is equivalent to having eight hours' jet lag every time they have a weekend off.

Such workers will not be able to establish a normal circadian body rhythm as they have an irregular sleep time and the circadian information obtained from their exposure to daylight conflicts with that from the timing of their sleep periods. It is not surprising that many have difficulty initiating and maintaining sleep during such cycles. Some seem to cope with these shifts much better than others, and there are genuine inter-individual variations in tolerance. Older people have greater difficulty adjusting to shifts[7,8] and those over 45 years old should be given the option of daytime working where possible.

Shift workers report short and interrupted sleep, chronic sleepiness and fatigue and have a high rate of inaccuracy at work.[9] Many will admit to falling asleep recurrently at work. These features of shift workers, sometimes combined with excessive work periods, probably contributed to some major recent accidents, including those involving the space shuttle *Challenger*, the Three Mile Island nuclear powerplant, the *Exxon Valdiz*[10] and to the Chernobyl disaster.[11] On a more everyday – but equally worrying – level, many night shift workers, up to 95 per cent in one series,[12] report road accidents or near accidents when driving to and from work. Doctors working at night report[13] falling asleep at the wheel significantly more often than those working by day (49 per cent versus 13 per cent; $p<0.001$).

The effects of shift work are not limited to performance but also extend to general health. Shift workers are reported to have higher rates of ischaemic heart disease, peptic ulcer and gastrointestinal symptoms than day workers.[14,15] It is not clear, however, whether this relates only to the reportedly higher rates of smoking in shift workers.

Treatment of individuals experiencing insomnia or problems with performance or sleepiness while working a shift system is often difficult, as they usually have no direct control over their shift pattern. Furthermore, changing to a permanent day job is rarely considered a realistic option. They should be encouraged to sleep for a normal duration and as far as possible at the same time of day during the different shifts – this will obviously not be feasible for those on a fully rotating shift pattern. They should avoid the temptation to burn the candle at both ends to the detriment of their health by participating in too many social activities that coincide with their usual sleeping time. Therapy with hypnotic drugs should be avoided.

Treatment with bright lights has been trialled in some shift workers with success in terms of obtaining a more rapid phase shift, better subjective sleep and improved mood.[16,17] However, it is not yet clear whether this results in improved work performance or alertness.[18] Although treatment with light boxes may not be currently practical for routine use in large numbers of shiftworkers, this approach is worth trying around shift changes in individuals who are particularly troubled by sleep-related problems when they alter their shifts.

Those planning shift work regimes need to be fully aware of the potentially detrimental effects on work performance and health. There is some evidence that rotating shifts should have slow cycle lengths, with workers spending at least a week in each shift, and that the shifts should be progressively delayed when changed, so moving from morning to late to night shift.[19] Both approaches tend to produce stabilization of the circadian rhythm.[20]

Useful review

- Akerstedt, T. (1998) Shift work and disturbed sleep/wakefulness. *Sleep Medicine Reviews*, **2**, 117–28.

Jet lag

Jet lag is a complex condition in which rapid travel across time zones is associated with asynchrony between the body's circadian clock and the actual local time. The sensations experienced are usually a combination of the results of this asynchrony and of sleep deprivation which is almost universal in such travellers. The sleep loss on flights may be compounded by poor-quality sleep resulting from uncomfortable sleeping posture, trying to sleep in an unusual environment and sometimes by alcohol excess. Up to a third of people deny they experience jet lag but the remainder will admit to difficulty getting to sleep after an eastward flight, wakening early after a westward flight, disturbed sleep, daytime sleepiness, difficulty concentrating, irritability, anorexia and nocturia. Whilst these symptoms may be a minor inconvenience at the start and end of trips for holidaymakers, they may seriously impair the ability to make appropriate decisions for businessmen, pilots and aircrew.

DECREASING JET LAG

The principle measures are:

- **Where possible do not change your time sleep times.** For short trips it may be possible not to shift your sleep times and go to bed and get up at the same times – by your home clock – as you would normally do. This often means missing evening social events – when flying westwards – or early morning functions – when flying eastwards – but for 24–48-hour trips can totally avoid any jet lag problems.
- **Obtain adequate sleep.** Daytime flights should be used where possible to minimize sleep loss. During overnight flights every effort should be made

to sleep as much as possible. Travelling business or first class and the use of earplugs and eyeshades may help, and consideration should be given to missing meals served during the time available for sleep. Alcohol and caffeine are deleterious to sleep quality, especially after large quantities, and ingestion should be moderated. On arrival in the new time zone judicious use of short naps, terminated by an alarm clock, may be useful in improving alertness and concentration,[21] but care must be taken not to nap late in the day as this will decrease the drive to sleep at night. Short-acting hypnotic drugs used on overnight flights and for a few nights after arrival[22] may help. However, the risks of drug-induced sleepiness carrying over into the next day have to be taken into account, particularly for short flights followed by important meetings or driving.

- **Optimize light exposure**. Light can alter the circadian clock and benefit jet lag.[23] The ideal timing of light exposure is debated but the most important component is to be exposed to bright light during the daytime for the new time zone and avoid bright light at other times. This usually means maximizing the exposure to light early in the day after flying eastwards and late in the day after flying westwards.
- **Take exercise**. Exercise both improves sleep quality[24] and has a minor effect on entraining circadian rhythms, night-time exercise delaying the circadian clock.[4]
- **Consider use of melatonin**. There are several controlled studies showing that melatonin at the local bedtime for a few nights after arrival is better than placebo in reducing jet lag symptoms.[25,26] However, melatonin has hypnotic properties[6] and there are no comparative studies against conventional short-acting hypnotic agents. In addition, in many parts of the world melatonin is not available or, worse, is not of standardized production or purity. Further, the long-term effects are unknown. Thus I would not recommend melatonin use for jet lag at present.

As well as trying to reduce jet lag, it is important that the traveller tries to ensure key meetings or decisions are timed to periods of maximal alertness. Thus, for trips westwards critical meetings should be held in the morning on local time, and on trips eastwards, in the afternoon or evening.

Useful review

- Haimov, I., Arendt, J. (1999) The prevention and treatment of jet lag. *Sleep Medicine Reviews*, **3**, 229–40.

Phase alteration syndromes

Some individuals develop alterations of their circadian system which result in changes in the timing of their sleep–wake cycle,[27] with either phase advance or delay (Figure 7.2). This often starts as a self-inflicted or work-caused change in sleep time, but then becomes self-perpetuating when the original motivation for altered sleep times ceases. For example, students may choose to work regularly into the early hours of the morning and then become set in a pattern of sleep onset in the early hours of the morning. Others may chose to go to bed late in order to maximize recreation. Shift workers may similarly adopt altered sleep schedules as a coping strategy, which then become fixed and tiresome once they stop working shifts. In others no precipitant can be found and endogenous factors may drive the phase alteration.

Figure 7.2
Sleep times in normal subjects and in individuals with phase advance and phase delay syndromes.

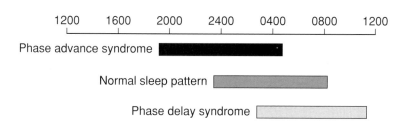

The key aspects of making these diagnoses are taking a clear history of patients' usual sleep onset and final wakening times and of the quality of nocturnal sleep. Asking patients to complete a sleep diary over a few weeks may be helpful (Chapter 6). Actimetric documentation of actual sleep times is often helpful both for diagnosis (Figure 7.3) and for following the effects of treatment. The diagnostic criteria are:

● **Phase delay/sleep onset insomnia:** (1) Normal or late bedtime with more than 45 minutes' sleep onset latency; (2) Few awakenings throughout the night with less than 30 minutes' wake throughout the night; (3) Late

Figure 7.3
Activity monitoring results over a two-week period in a 16-year-old girl with phase delay syndrome. Each 24-hour period is double-plotted so that consecutive nights are vertically above each other in the centre of the plot. The results show the usual time of sleep onset was between 0300 and 0400 and of awakening 1200 to 1400 hours.

Rhythm watch
Actogram printout

User identification
Start date   21-Sep   Start time   11:50
Subject age   Subject sex   F   Epoch length 0.5 (Mins)
Vertical Scale   1700   Zero Clip 0

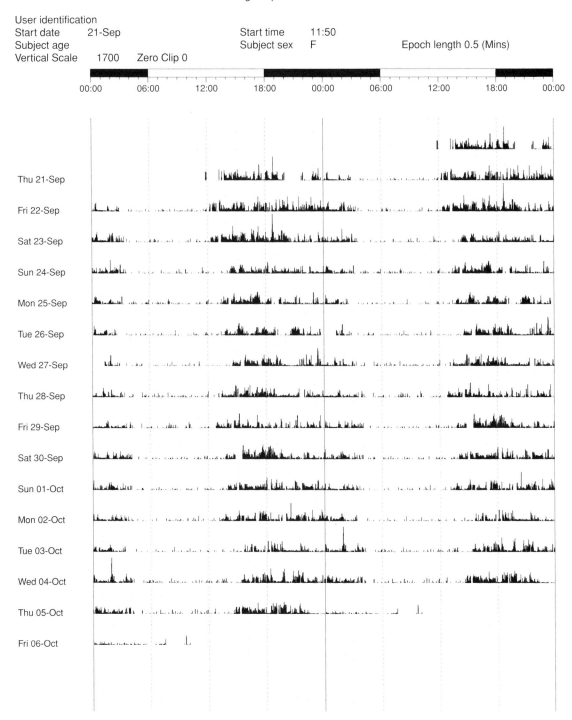

final wakening or reported insufficient sleep; (4) Absence of other causes of insomnia.

- **Phase advancement/early morning wakening insomnia**: (1) Early bedtime with rapid (less than 15 minute) sleep onset; (2) Difficulty maintaining sleep later in the night (after about 5 am); (3) Alert in morning but increasing sleepiness in the evening; (4) Absence of other causes of insomnia.

TREATMENT OF PHASE ALTERATION SYNDROMES

Considerable progress has been made in recent years in the treatment of phase alteration problems with light therapy[28] and melatonin. Phase delay syndrome – when sleep onset and final awakening are later than desirable – can be treated either with bright light therapy in the morning or melatonin at bedtime. Phase advance syndrome – too early sleep onset and final awakening – can be usefully treated with either bright light therapy in the evening or melatonin in the morning.

Early morning bright light advances the body clock both in normal subjects[29] and in insomniacs with phase alteration syndromes.[30] Placebo- (dim red light) controlled trials have shown that morning bright light therapy results in significantly better reported sleep duration in patients with phase delay insomnia.[31]

An alternative to light therapy is melatonin, although the safety of this is not well documented and so it is not currently recommended. However, for phase delay insomnia, melatonin taken two hours before the intended bedtime can be beneficial and, for phase advancement insomnia, melatonin late in the night or in the early morning may be helpful.

Appropriate therapy plans for patients with **phase delay** and sleep onset insomnia therefore are:

- Avoid sleeping in the morning by setting an alarm to seven hours after usual sleep onset.
- Bright light stimulation (>2000 lux) for at least an hour each morning for at least seven days followed by two to three mornings per week over the next four weeks. Initially, light therapy should be started about seven hours after patients' usual sleep onset time, and then the time of therapy should be gradually drifted towards a normal final wakening time. The light should be placed well within the field of view and ideally some of the time should be spent directly gazing at the light.
- Avoid bright light in the evening.
- Morning exercise and a hot bath may be helpful in resetting the circadian clock, as may morning caffeine.

- Melatonin 1–5 mg orally two hours before usual sleep onset time may be a useful adjunct in some patients, but should not be used for more than one week.

For those with **phase advancement** and early morning wakening insomnia:

- Bright light stimulation (>2000 lux) for at least two hours each evening ending at least one hour after the normal time of sleep onset. Light should be used nightly for at least seven days and then two to three times per week for the next four weeks. Often placing the light box just beneath the line between the patient and the TV is a good method of achieving compliance.
- Avoid bright lights in the morning.
- Late evening hot baths/showers may be helpful. Morning exercise should be avoided, evening exercise is of debatable value.
- Melatonin is not normally recommended, but has been used at low doses (<2 mg) late in the sleep period, but should be restricted to seven days' therapy or less.

Useful reviews

- Campbell, S.S., Murphy, P.J., van den Heuvel, C.J., Roberts, M.L., Stauble, T.N. (1999) Etiology and treatment of intrinsic circadian rhythm sleep disorders. *Sleep Medicine Reviews*, **3**, 179–200.
- Richardson, G., Tate, B. (2000) Hormonal and pharmacological manipulation of the circadian clock: recent developments and future strategies. *Sleep*, **23** (Suppl. 3), S77–S85.
- Skene, D.J., Lockley, S.W., Arendt, J. (1999) Use of melatonin in the treatment of phase shift and sleep disorders. *Adv. Exp. Med. Biol.*, **467**, 79–84.

References

1 Moore, R.Y., Lenn, N.J. (1972) A retinohypothalamic projection in the rat. *J. Comp. Neurol.*, **146**, 1–14.
2 Boivin, D.B., Czeisler, C.A. (1998) Resetting of circadian melatonin and cortisol rhythms in humans by ordinary room light. *Neuroreport*, **9**, 779–82.

3   Boivin, D.B., Duffy, J.F., Kronauer, R.E., Czeisler, C.A. (1996) Dose-response relationships for resetting of human circadian clock by light. *Nature*, **379**, 540–2.

4   Van Reeth, O., Sturis, J., Byrne, M.M., Blackman, J.D., L'Hermite-Baleriaux, M., Leproult, R. *et al.* (1994) Nocturnal exercise phase delays circadian rhythms of melatonin and thyrotropin secretion in normal men. *Am. J. Physiol.*, **266**, E964–E974.

5   Zaidan, R., Geoffriau, M., Brun, J., Taillard, J., Bureau, C., Chazot, G. *et al.* (1994) Melatonin is able to influence its secretion in humans: description of a phase-response curve. *Neuroendocrinology*, **60**, 105–12.

6   Sack, R.L., Hughes, R.J., Edgar, D.M., Lewy, A.J. (1997) Sleep-promoting effects of melatonin: at what dose, in whom, under what conditions, and by what mechanisms? *Sleep,* **20**, 908–15.

7   Harma, M., Suvanto, S., Partinen, M. (1994) The effect of four-day round trip flights over 10 time zones on the sleep–wakefulness patterns of airline flight attendants. *Ergonomics*, **37**, 1461–78.

8   Reid, K., Dawson, D. (2001) Comparing performance on a simulated 12 hour shift rotation in young and older subjects. *Occup. Environ. Med.*, **58**, 58–62.

9   Bjerner, B., Holm, A., Swensson, A. (1955) Diurnal variation of mental performance. A study of three-shift workers. *Br. J. Ind. Med.*, **12**, 103–10.

10 National Commission on Sleep Disorders Research. (1993) *Wake Up America: A National Sleep Alert.* Washington: US Government Printing Office.

11 Mitler, M.M., Carskadon, M.A., Czeisler, C.A., Dement, W.C., Dinges, D.F., Graeber, R.C. (1988) Catastrophes, sleep, and public policy: consensus report. *Sleep*, **11**, 100–9.

12 Novak, R.D., Auvil-Novak, S.E. (1996) Focus group evaluation of night nurse shiftwork difficulties and coping strategies. *Chronobiol. Int.*, **13**, 457–63.

13 Marcus, C.L., Loughlin, G.M. (1996) Effect of sleep deprivation on driving safety in housestaff. *Sleep*, **19**, 763–6.

14 Alfredsson, L., Karasek, R., Theorell, T. (1982) Myocardial infarction risk and psychosocial work environment: an analysis of the male Swedish working force. *Soc. Sci. Med.*, **16**, 463–7.

15 Koller, M. (1983) Health risks related to shift work. An example of time-contingent effects of long-term stress. *Int. Arch. Occup. Environ. Health*, **53**, 59–75.

16 Stewart, K.T., Hayes, B.C., Eastman, C.I. (1995) Light treatment for NASA shiftworkers. *Chronobiol. Int.*, **12**, 141–51.

17 Eastman, C.I., Liu, L., Fogg, L.F. (1995) Circadian rhythm adaptation to simulated night shift work: effect of nocturnal bright-light duration. *Sleep*, **18**, 399–407.

18 Campbell, S.S. (1995) Effects of timed bright-light exposure on shift-work adaptation in middle-aged subjects. *Sleep*, **18**, 408–16.

19 Barton, J., Folkard, S., Smith, L., Poole, C.J. (1994) Effects on health of a change from a delaying to an advancing shift system. *Occup. Environ. Med.*, **51**, 749–55.

20 Czeisler, C.A., Moore-Ede, M.C., Coleman, R.H. (1982) Rotating shift work schedules that disrupt sleep are improved by applying circadian principles. *Science*, **217**, 460–3.

21 Stone, B.M., Turner, C. (1997) Promoting sleep in shiftworkers and intercontinental travelers. *Chronobiol. Int.*, **14**, 133–43.

22 Redfern, P.H. (1992) Can pharmacological agents be used effectively in the alleviation of jet-lag? *Drugs*, **43**, 146–53.

23 Samel, A., Wegmann, H.M. (1997) Bright light: a countermeasure for jet lag? *Chronobiol. Int.*, **14**, 173–83.

24 Shapiro, C.M., Warren, P.M., Trinder, J., Paxton, S.J., Oswald, I., Flenley, D.C. *et al.* (1984) Fitness facilitates sleep. *Eur. J. Appl. Physiol. Occup. Physiol.*, **53**, 1–4.

25 Arendt, J. (1998) Jet-lag. *Lancet*, **351**, 293–4.

26 Arendt, J. (2000) Melatonin, circadian rhythms, and sleep. *N. Engl. J. Med.*, **343**, 1114–16.

27 Roehrs, T., Salin-Pascual, R., Merlotti, L., Rosenthal, L., Roth, T. (1996) Phase advance in moderately sleepy and alert normals. *Sleep*, **19**, 417–22.

28 Chesson, A.L., Littner, M., Davila, D., Anderson, W.M., Grigg-Damberger, M., Hartse, K. *et al.* (1999) Practice parameters for the use of light therapy in the treatment of sleep disorders. Standards of Practice Committee, American Academy of Sleep Medicine. *Sleep*, **22**, 641–60.

29 Dawson, D., Lack, L., Morris, M. (1993) Phase resetting of the human circadian pacemaker with use of a single pulse of bright light. *Chronobiol. Int.*, **10**, 94–102.

30 Lack, L., Wright, H. (1993) The effect of evening bright light in delaying the circadian rhythms and lengthening the sleep of early morning awakening insomniacs. *Sleep*, **16**, 436–43.

31 Lack, L.C., Gibbon, S., Schumaker, K., Wright, H. (1994) Comparison of bright and placebo light treatments for morning insomnia. *Sleep Res.*, **23**, 278.

Miscellaneous sleep disorders

Night terrors

Night terrors are characterized by a sudden arousal from sleep, usually with a very loud scream followed by a sensation of terror associated with tachycardia, tachypnoea and sweating. Often there may be a significant motor component which may cause difficulty differentiating night terrors from sleepwalking.

AETIOLOGY

The arousal is usually from stage 3 or 4 (slow wave) sleep, although occasionally episodes may start from Stage 2 sleep. In adults, stages 3 and 4 sleep is mainly found during the first sleep cycle and thus night terrors usually occur in the first 90 minutes of sleep. In children, stages 3 and 4 sleep episodes continue later into the night than in adults and so night terrors may be spread over the first half of the night.

In most cases there is a family history, with 96 per cent reporting other members of the family who had night terrors or sleep walking in one series.[1] The genetic basis for this is unknown.

EPIDEMIOLOGY

Children have a far higher frequency of night terrors than adults, with childhood rates of one to six per cent[1,2] in comparison to well under one per cent in adults. The peak age for the condition is five to seven years. Most children tend to grow out of the problem in around four years. However, attacks can be persistent and most adults with terrors report having episodes since childhood, although occasionally they may arise *de novo* in adult life.

CLINICAL FEATURES

Sleep terrors start suddenly with a loud shriek, often referred to as blood-curdling. Sufferers are often found sitting in bed screaming with a look of extreme panic, eyes bulging and heart racing. They often thrash around and kick and make unintelligible attempts at speech. They will not respond to voice, touch or reassurance. Sometimes they may leap out of bed and run about, including fleeing from the bedroom. Self-injury is common during such extreme events, as they run into furniture, doors and even through windows. The episodes last from a few seconds up to 15 minutes or so. After the attack subsides the sufferer usually appears confused and still agitated. However, patients often exhibit a striking ability to fall back to sleep rapidly after such events, even mid-conversation. In the morning, they usually have no memory of these events despite their alarming nature.

Attacks normally occur once or twice per week initially, although occasionally several attacks may occur within a single night. The frequency of attacks tends to decline gradually.

DIFFERENTIAL DIAGNOSIS

Simple sleepwalking needs to be differentiated, particularly as many night terror sufferers also sleepwalk. Differentiating features include the initiating scream, the profound terror and the usually purposeless movement. Nightmares can also cause confusion, but again the characteristic scream and marked panic usually suffice to distinguish terrors from nightmares. In addition, nightmares, rather than terrors, are suggested by the ease of arousing from an episode, rapid return to alertness, recall of 'nightmare' content, lack of confusion and disorientation after the event.

DIAGNOSIS

In most cases, a confident clinical diagnosis can be made. However, occasionally overnight polysomnography is required. One of the problems with polysomnography is that events do not occur every night and it is common to record several nights before an attack is observed – an inconvenient and expensive undertaking. Thus I rarely perform polysomnography in such patients. Home video recording is generally more useful as it can be repeated until attacks occur. Sometimes this may be combined with home sleep stage recording. Patients with sleep terrors may show suggestive brief recurrent arousals from stages 3 and 4 sleep even in the absence of a terror attack. Full-blown attacks arising from stages 3 and 4 associated with tachycardia and tachypnoea are the hallmark of diagnosis in the difficult case.[3]

TREATMENT

Parents should be advised to stay as calm as possible during attacks and only to restrain the child if there is an immediate threat of self-injury. The bedroom environment should be made as safe as possible with objects which may cause injury removed, and doors and windows locked. A regular bedtime routine may reduce attacks in some patients, whereas overtiredness may predispose to terrors. Parents should be reassured that the attacks will subside with time leaving no long-term sequelae. They should also be informed that trying to wake sufferers during attacks is rarely helpful. Parents and siblings should be as supportive as possible. Both should be aware that the victim will have no recollection of the events and that anxiety is commonly the patient's reaction to the family's response to the episodes.

These measures alone will be sufficient in most children with night terrors, but when events persist into adolescence or occur *de novo* in adolescence a psychogenic predisposition should be sought and treated as appropriate.[4] Episodes may be suppressed in some adolescents and adults by benzodiazepine therapy.[5] Hypnotics are thought to act by suppressing the arousal response. There is, however, a high rate of relapse especially during periods of stress.

Sleepwalking

Sleep walking, or somnabulism, occurs suddenly and without warning usually within the first three hours after sleep onset. Children usually grow out of the behaviour.

AETIOLOGY

The high prevalence in early childhood and the resolution with puberty suggests that neuro-maturational factors are important.[6] High-voltage slow wave activity on the electroencephalogram has been reported to persist into later childhood in sleepwalkers than in others.

Episodes may be induced in predisposed children by stimulating them during slow wave sleep.[7] The frequency of sleepwalking can also be increased by sleep deprivation, physical fatigue or fever.[6] Sedatives, hypnotic drugs and alcohol may also induce attacks.

Although psychopathology is rare in children who sleepwalk, it is important in sleepwalking adults. Approximately 75 per cent of adult sleepwalkers have been said to have personality disorders,[8] but not those who used to sleepwalk as children.

Sleepwalking is also more common in children with migraine[9,10] and with Tourette's syndrome.[11]

EPIDEMIOLOGY

Fifteen to 30 per cent of healthy children will sleep walk at some stage with approximately three per cent having done so often.[12,13] Episodes usually start in early childhood with a peak prevalence before puberty[13] and most will have grown out of sleepwalking by the age of 15 years. About one per cent of adults sleepwalk and most will have continued to sleepwalk from childhood. Sleepwalking after the age of 60 is rare.

Prevalence is equal in males and females. There is a strong familial tendency with 80 per cent of sleepwalkers having family members who either sleepwalked or had night terrors.[8] There is a higher concordance in monozygotic than dizygotic twins.[14] Sleeptalking is about six times more common in sleepwalkers than non-sleepwalkers. As there is a familial trait in sleep talking, some believe the mechanism of these two conditions may be linked.

CLINICAL FEATURES

Episodes usually start with subjects suddenly sitting up in bed, often with a vacant facial expression and unawareness of their surroundings. They then get out of bed and walk around the room or out of the room, often in a clumsy and purposeless manner. However, complex movements can be achieved and eating, drinking, talking on the telephone and playing musical instruments have been reported. Sleeptalking may occur, but the extreme shouts typical of night terrors are unusual.

Although subjects can usually walk around obstacles without difficulty, in other ways they show little awareness of their environment. However, seemingly purposeful behaviour can prove very dangerous with sufferers having fallen from building, smashed through windows and doors and even reported to have crashed cars[15,16] and committed murder.[17] Calling the sufferers' name typically evokes no purposeful response and attempting to shake them into wakefulness will often meet limited success or produce a confused half-asleep individual.

Most episodes start within three hours of sleep onset, during the time that stage 3/4 sleep is more prevalent. Attacks usually last around 10 minutes whereupon subjects returns to bed and rapidly fall asleep. More than one episode in a night is rare. Unless awoken during the episode, there will be no recall of the event in the morning.

DIFFERENTIAL DIAGNOSIS

Sleepwalking may need to be differentiated from sleep terrors, REM sleep behavioural disorders and complex partial seizures, although usually the clinical features are sufficiently characteristic to allow a confident diagnosis to be made.

The loud shouts and intense autonomic responses of sleep terrors allow distinction to be made. REM sleep behavioural disorder typically occurs in the elderly often in association with neurological disease and attacks happen later in the night. Complex partial seizures may also occur during wakefulness, are more frequently associated with automatism and awakening and may happen throughout the night, often during REM sleep.

DIAGNOSIS

A confident clinical diagnosis of sleepwalking can almost always be made. In very exceptional cases where doubt exists about authenticity or diagnosis, polysomnographic recording either in the sleep laboratory or at home may be required. This may show the episodes arising from the first sleep cycle and preceded by bursts of slow waves. During sleep walks the EEG tends to be obscured by movement artefacts but features of non-REM sleep or alpha rhythm may be seen.

TREATMENT

The only measures usually needed are a combination of reassurance of all involved, recognition that subjects almost always grow out of the condition at puberty and the removal of objects which could be hazardous. When found during an episode subjects should be gently led back to bed. Generally, no reference should be made to the episode in the morning in an attempt to minimize anxiety.

Occasionally doors and window catches may need modifying for safety and, in some circumstances, bars may need to be placed on windows and special locks on exterior doors. Some will need to request ground floor rooms in hotels for safety reasons. Subjects should avoid sleep deprivation whenever possible, and thus adults significantly troubled by sleepwalking should not work rotating night/day shifts.

Wakening sufferers just before the usual time of sleepwalking can abolish episodes, presumably by disrupting the sleep cycle[18] and may sometimes be helpful. Rarely, therapy with benzodiazepines may be indicated, particularly when episodes are potentially life-threatening or when sufferers may be away from home and concerned about the responses of others to the episodes.

However, as benzodiazepines can increase attacks in some patients they should be used with caution.

Those who develop sleepwalking *de novo* in adult life should be assessed for psychological/psychiatric illness and treated accordingly.

REM sleep behaviour disorders

In 1986, Schenck and colleagues[19] reported four patients with vigorous movements and dream-like activities in association with REM sleep and coined the term 'REM sleep behaviour disorder'. This, they suggested, was a manifestation of an age-related degenerative condition affecting REM motor function.

AETIOLOGY

Approximately 60 per cent of cases of REM sleep behaviour disorder are associated with a known neurological disease and the remaining 40 per cent are idiopathic. There is a wide range of associated neurological conditions (Table 8.1). However, the precise site of lesions which results in the condition is not known. The pedunculopontine nucleus seems critical for the interaction of locomotor and sleep–wake mechanisms.[20] This nucleus through connections to the thalamus may determine both the EEG desynchronization and the generation of pontogeniculate waves during REM sleep. Projections to the substantia nigra may explain the high rate of REM sleep behaviour disorder in Parkinsonism.[21] However, these suggested mechanisms are not proven.

Table 8.1

Neurological conditions associated with REM sleep behaviour disorder

Parkinsonism
Dementia
Olivopontine cerebellar degeneration
Shy–Drager syndrome
Narcolepsy
Cerebrovascular disease
Multiple sclerosis
Astrocytoma
Alcohol abuse

Drugs:
    imipramine
    monoamine oxidase inhibitors
    amphetamine

(Data from Schenck and Mahowald[22] and Sforza, Kreiger and Petiau[24].)

EPIDEMIOLOGY

The prevalence of the condition is unknown. In one series of patients with motor disorders during sleep, REM-related movement disorders accounted for 31 per cent of 170 cases, but this may be skewed by the referrals due to authors' expertise in this area.[22]

Most cases start after the age of 50 years, although in a minority there may be a history of sleeptalking and sleep-related movements going back to childhood or early adult life. Nearly 90 per cent of sufferers are male.[23]

CLINICAL FEATURES

Most patients with REM sleep behavioural disorder present with the combination of vigorous motor activity accompanying vivid dreams. The movement often results in repeated injury, over half reporting repetitive bruising, and others cuts and fractures. The lengths that sufferers go to protect themselves – erecting pillow barricades or sleeping on a mattress on the floor – are testimony to the serious and recurrent nature of the condition.

Acting out of dreams starts at least 90 minutes after sleep onset, when the first REM sleep cycle begins, and up to the final morning awakening. The dreams are usually repetitive and stereotyped, often patients are trying to fight back or flee from an attack, but unfortunately harm themselves or their partner in the attempt. Sleeptalking may or may not be intelligible. Patients may yell, laugh, swear, punch, kick, jump out of bed or even run away. Although jerky limb movements may occur every night, major movement episodes usually take place between four times per night and once a fortnight. Patients rarely complain of sleep disruption, being more concerned with injury. Indeed, awakenings when they occur are more often due to the attentions of patients' partners trying to end episodes rather than to spontaneous arousal. When they are awoken, there is a rapid return to alertness, excellent recall of the offending dream and rapid return to normal behaviour. The violent nocturnal behaviour is generally totally out of character for the patient's daytime persona.

DIFFERENTIAL DIAGNOSIS

Potential confusion may occur with a variety of disorders including:

- Sleepwalking.
- Sleep terrors.
- Sleep apnoea/hypopnoea syndrome.

- Periodic limb movement disorder (PLMD).
- Nocturnal epilepsy.
- Malingering.

In most patients the majority of the above diagnoses can be readily differentiated from REM sleep behavioural disorder by obtaining a clear history from the patient and the bed partner, particularly of the timing of the attacks, the type of movements which occur and the level of consciousness during episodes. Differentiation from nocturnal epilepsy may be the most difficult, REM sleep behaviour disorder being suggested by organized and quasi-purposeful motor activity and the absence of tonic–clonic movements. The delay in onset of abnormal movements until after at least an hour of sleep helps to differentiate from PLMD and other non-REM sleep parasomnias. However, a firm diagnosis will require investigation.

DIAGNOSIS

The key to the diagnosis of REM sleep behavioural disorder is the combination of a history of a sleep behaviour which is:

- Potentially or actually harmful.
- Disrupts sleep.
- Annoys the patient or bed partner.

In the North American context diagnosis is accompanied by polysomnographic evidence of:

- Excessive chin EMG during REM sleep.
- Excessive twitching of chin or limb EMG during REM sleep.

Videotaping during polysomnography can also be useful, demonstrating REM-related movements which may be typified by excessive limb or body jerking, complex nature and/ or violence. It is important to note that sleeptalking, yelling and nightmares have been also reported during non-REM sleep in patients with REM-related behaviour disorders.

In reality, the correct clinical features in an older man allows a confident clinical diagnosis to be made and I rarely resort to polysomnography unless there is diagnostic uncertainty or therapeutic difficulty.

In view of the association with a range of central nervous system (CNS) disorders, a neurological opinion should be sought in patients with new neurological abnormality suggested on either history or examination – at least in younger patients.

TREATMENT

Benzodiazepines are the treatment of choice and are effective in 90 per cent of patients within a week. Most studies have used clonazepam, initially taking 0.5 mg two hours before bedtime. After early total suppression of attacks, abnormal motor activity may recur, but the frequency and severity of attacks is reduced compared with prior to commencing treatment. After at least four years' therapy, the mean dose of clonazepam producing satisfactory clinical responses was 1 mg.[22] Anecdotal reports have indicated that tricyclic antidepressants – a logical way to reduce REM sleep – and carbemazepine may be of benefit.

Useful review

- Sforza, E., Krieger, J., Petiau, C. (1997) REM sleep behavior disorder: clinical and physiopathological findings. *Sleep Medicine Reviews*, **1**, 57–69.

PLMD treatment

Previously called nocturnal myoclonus, PLMD consists of movement of one or both legs repetitively during sleep. This phenomenon is very common, particularly in the elderly, but it is unclear how often it causes symptoms.

AETIOLOGY

The neurological mechanism behind this disorder is unknown. The marked periodicity of the movements strongly suggest the existence of a CNS pacemaker. Studies both during sleep and coma have suggested a 20–40 second periodicity in respiration, heart rate blood pressure and EEG arousal.[25] The periodicity of these variables is similar to that of PLMs and may occur synchronous with PLMs. These observations suggest the presence of a subcortical pacemaker perhaps regulated by rhythmic fluctuations of the reticular system.

EPIDEMIOLOGY

The prevalence of periodic limb movement during sleep is closely related to age. It is very rare below the age of 30, occurs in around five per cent of normal subjects aged 30–50 years, about 30 per cent in those over 50 and nearly 50 per cent in subjects over 65.[26,27]

CLINICAL FEATURES

Periodic limb movements (PLMs) are repetitive rhythmic dorsiflexions of the ankle with extension of the big toe sometimes associated with flexion of the knee and hip. Each movement lasts 0.5–5 seconds, and the movements are repeated every 20–40 seconds. Movements tend to be more frequent in the first half of the night but often occur throughout non-REM sleep.

Conditions which have been associated with PLMD include restless legs syndrome *(see below),* diabetes, uraemia, anaemia, leukaemia, chronic lung disease, rheumatoid arthritis and fibromyositis. However, many of these conditions are common in middleaged and elderly people and it is not clear whether the frequency of PLMs is increased in all of them compared to an age-matched normal population.

DIFFERENTIAL DIAGNOSIS

PLMs needs to be differentiated from other motor events during sleep.

Hypnic jerks, or sleep starts, occur at sleep onset and are a normal physiological phenomenon. They are major jerks which may involve much of the body and do not have a rhythmic pattern. Hypnic jerks cease once sleep is established.

L-dopa can induce body jerks, but these tend to be infrequent, perhaps three to 30 per night, thus allowing easy differentiation from PLMs.

DIAGNOSIS

Periodic limb movements are scored from polysomnography traces provided they are part of a run of four or more consecutive movements lasting 0.5–5 seconds, with an inter-movement interval of 5–90 seconds. More than five PLMs per hour slept is often considered to be pathological.[28]

TREATMENT

There are no adequately powered randomized controlled trials investigating the benefits of any therapy in PMLD without restless legs.[29] However, L-dopa is usually regarded as the treatment of choice.[28,30] Usual practice is to start with 50 mg orally half an hour before bed, the dose being increased thereafter until symptomatic control is achieved. Often a dosage of around

200 mg at night in conjunction with a dopa decarboxylase inhibitor is required. Other agents which may be helpful include benzodiazepines[31] – which may mainly suppress the arousals rather than the leg movements – bromocriptine and carbamazepine.

PLMs should not be treated unless they are associated with sleep-related symptoms. Controlled trials are needed to establish whether treating PLMs in patients with insomnia or hypersomnolence who are found to have PLMs is of clinical benefit. At present it seems reasonable to treat patients with severe sleep maintenance insomnia or marked hypersomnolence in whom PLMs are the only abnormality found.

Useful review

- Hening, W., Allen, R., Earley, C., Kushida, C., Picchietti, D., Silber, M. (1999) The treatment of restless legs syndrome and periodic limb movement disorder. An American Academy of Sleep Medicine Review. *Sleep,* **22**, 970–99.

Restless legs syndrome

CLINICAL FEATURES

Restless legs syndrome (RLS) is characterized by paraesthesia or dysaesthesia of the legs, an intense urge to move them and motor restlessness. Patients may complain about unpleasant creeping sensations deep in the legs and a compelling desire to move the legs, flexing, stretching and crossing them repeatedly. Occasionally, the upper limbs can also be affected. The symptoms tend to become worse at bedtime and can cause difficulty initiating sleep. All the symptoms are worse in the evening or night.[30] About 90 per cent of patients with RLS have PLMs during sleep.

RLS patients have low iron levels,[32] a finding is of considerable pathophysiological interest, but its clinical significance is unclear. A placebo-controlled trial of iron therapy for 12 weeks showed no clinical benefit.[33]

EPIDEMIOLOGY

The condition affects approximately two per cent of the population, men and women equally.

DIAGNOSIS

This is a clinical diagnosis. Sleep studies are not diagnostic as approximately 10 per cent of patients do not have PLMs. Renal failure, iron deficiency and, where appropriate, pregnancy should be sought as possible causes.

TREATMENT

There are placebo-controlled studies showing benefit in patients with the RLS from L-dopa[34,35] or pergolide[36] in terms of reducing PLMs and improving subjective sleep quality.

Useful review

- Hening, W., Allen, R., Earley, C., Kushida, C., Picchietti, D., Silber, M. (1999) Treatment of restless legs syndrome and periodic limb movement disorder. An American-Academy of Sleep Medicine Review. *Sleep*, **22**, 970–99.

Snoring

Snoring is caused by the upper airway narrowing during sleep and the disturbed flow causing audible vibrations. The mechanism for this are identical to those detailed in Chapter 2 for obstructive sleep apnoea/hypopnoea syndrome (OSAHS), although the extent of narrowing is less in snoring than in apnoea or hypopnoea.

Approximately 40 per cent of men and 30 per cent of women are said by their partners to snore.[37–40] The noise of snoring can be extremely loud and has been measured as equivalent to a pneumatic road drill. The main predisposing factors to snoring are:

- Age – middle-aged or elderly.
- Overweight.
- Alcohol.
- Retrognathia.
- Nasal blockage.
- Smoking.[41]

It is not clear to what extent snoring has any medical consequences. The reported associations with ischaemic heart disease, stroke and hypertension could be due either to co-morbidities, such as obesity and smoking, or to these associations being solely with OSAHS and not with the majority of snorers who are simple snorers.[42–44]

Before any treatment is planned the possibility of co-existing OSAHS should be considered at least by taking a careful history. Treatment of simple snoring is by losing weight, avoiding alcohol and stopping smoking where relevant. If these are not achieved or not relevant then the following may be considered.

MANDIBULAR REPOSITIONING SPLINTS

The treatment of choice of troublesome snoring is a mandibular repositioning splint (MRS) designed to hold the mandible forwards during sleep. These have been shown in randomized controlled trials to reduce snoring.[45] Further studies need to be performed to assess the optimal splint design.[46,47] Current data suggest that the aim of the MRS should be to advance the mandible to around 75 per cent of maximal protrusion.

SURGERY

Surgery designed to improve the nasal airway is disappointingly ineffective as a treatment of snoring.[48] Uvulopalatopharyngoplasty (UPPP; U3P) can change or even silence the noise but these effects may not be long-lasting, it does not prevent OSAHS and can make treatment of OSAHS if it develops – or was missed initially – difficult or impossible.[49] Surgery to the throat for snoring should not be performed unless an adequate sleep study has confirmed severe snoring – as there is a poor correlation between partner's complaints and objective measurements[50] – and excluded OSAHS. One of the major unknowns is how rapidly severe snorers without OSAHS progress to OSAHS. There is, however enough anecdotal evidence from new OSAHS patients that they have progressed from loud snorers to cause me to advise snorers that UPPP is not a sensible option at present.

RADIOFREQUENCY VOLUME REDUCTION

There has been a recent vogue for treating snoring with radiofrequency volume reduction of the tongue or soft palate – often referred to by the trade name of Somnoplasty. This may reduce snoring and sleep apnoea in the short term in uncontrolled studies.[51–53] However, there are doubts about the long-term efficacy.[54] Thus this treatment cannot be advised at present.

Central sleep apnoea

Central apnoeas are respiratory pauses caused by lack of respiratory effort. Central apnoeas occur occasionally in normal subjects, particularly at sleep onset and in REM sleep. Most recurrent central apnoea is found in the context of cardiac failure (page 233) or neurological disease, especially stroke (page 233), and spontaneous central sleep apnoea syndrome is rare, with sleep centres seeing at least 100 patients with OSAHS for every one with clinically significant spontaneous central sleep apnoea. These cases can be divided on the basis of their arterial PCO_2.

Hypercapnic central sleep apnoea occurs in conjunction with diminished ventilatory drive in Ondine's curse (central alveolar hypoventilation).[55] This may perhaps occur also with the obesity hypoventilation syndrome, but obstructive apnoeas are much more common in these patients, and in the grossly obese detecting continued respiratory effort is technically demanding *(see below)*.

Normocapnic spontaneous central sleep apnoea patients have a normal or low arterial PCO_2 when awake and brisk ventilatory responses to hypercapnia.[56] This combination results in these individuals breathing close to their apnoeic threshold for PCO_2 during sleep, which is compounded by cycles of arousal-induced hyperventilation and further hypocapnia.

CLINICAL FEATURES

Because of the rarity of spontaneous central sleep apnoea and of the uncertainty of diagnostic accuracy in early studies, the clinical features are poorly documented.[57–59] Many patients seem to present with sleep maintenance insomnia which is relatively unusual in OSAHS. Daytime sleepiness may occur.

INVESTIGATION

Many apnoeas previously labelled central because of no thoraco-abdominal movement are actually obstructive, identification of movement being particularly difficult in the very obese. Central apnoeas can only be identified with certainty if either oesophageal pressure[60] or respiratory muscle electromyography is recorded and absent during the events.

TREATMENT

Patients with underlying cardiac failure should have their failure treated appropriately and CPAP may also be tried *(see* Chapter 11). Those with spontaneous normocapnic central sleep apnoea may be successfully treated with acetazolamide.[58] In some patients CPAP is effective and there may be several reasons for this. First, some of those reported as having central sleep apnoea may have had OSAHS but been studied before the limitations of surface sensors for apnoea classification were clear. Second, in some patients with OSAHS, pharyngeal collapse initiates reflex inhibition of respiration and these episodes are prevented by CPAP.[61,62] Other treatment which may be tried include oxygen[63] and nocturnal nasal IPPV.

Bruxism

Grinding of the teeth during sleep – or bruxism – is usually brought to medical attention by irritated bed partners, but sometimes because of tooth wear, tooth hypersensitivity or pain. The condition is commonest in childhood when up to 20 per cent of children may grind their teeth, falling to around three per cent when 60 years old.[26] Usually bruxism is a primary problem, but occasionally it can arise secondary to drugs, including selective serotonin re-uptake inhibitors (SSRIs) and amphetamines, or in association with other conditions, including dyskinesias, Parkinson's disease and stroke.

DIAGNOSIS

The diagnosis can be made clinically from the story of the noise of teeth grinding or tapping during sleep and features of jaw discomfort, teeth sensitivity and tooth wear.

TREATMENT

There is no cure but explanation to all parties involved can help, especially reassurance that bruxism tends to get better with age. Advice on sleep hygiene and relaxation are often given, but there is no convincing controlled evidence of efficacy. An occlusal appliance, such as an athletic gum guard or specialized device, may help reduce tooth wear and noise. However, the long-term use of these devices is disappointing with less than 20 per cent of patients still using them at one year.[64] Benzodiazepines, antidepressants, L-dopa and propranolol have all been tried but with limited and poorly documented success rates.

Useful review

- Bader, G., Lavigne, G. (2000) Sleep bruxism; an overview of an oro-mandibular sleep movement disorder. *Sleep Medicine Reviews*, **4**, 27–43.

Enuresis

Bladder control matures at different rates in boys and girls and bedwetting after the age of five in girls and after age six in boys is considered enuresis. Thereafter, enuresis spontaneously remits at a rate of around 15 per cent of cases per annum, with less than one per cent persisting into adult life.

Enuretic children tend to have a lower birth weight, smaller stature and delayed developmental milestones, all suggesting that maturation is an important factor.[65] Psychological factors can also be important, especially in those who develop secondary enuresis having previously been dry for at least three months. Only a very small minority have any anatomical abnormality of the urinary tract. Diabetes mellitus should be excluded.

TREATMENT

Management is principally based on reassurance and support whilst awaiting spontaneous resolution. In a minority of subjects an alarm sensitive to bed-wetting may be used.[66] These are thought to work by conditioning the individual to waken before the alarm rings and then to get up and go to the toilet. Overall results are good with only around two per cent of enuretic children still bedwetting at age 14 years.[67]

Useful review

- Challamel, M.-J., Cochat, P. (1999) Enuresis: pathophysiology and treatment. *Sleep Medicine Reviews*, **3**, 313–24.

References

1 Kales, J.D., Kales, A., Soldatos, C.R., Caldwell, A.B., Charney, D.S., Martin, E.D. (1980) Night terrors. Clinical characteristics and personality patterns. *Arch. Gen. Psychiatry*, **37**, 1413–17.

2   Beltramini, A.U., Hertzig, M.E. (1983) Sleep and bedtime behavior in preschool-aged children. *Pediatrics,* **71**, 153–8.

3   Fisher, C., Kahn, E., Edwards, A., Davis, D.M. (1973) A psycho-physiological study of nightmares and night terrors. I. Physiological aspects of the stage 4 night terror. *J. Nerv. Ment. Dis.,* **157**, 75–98.

4   Kales, J.C., Cadieux, R.J., Soldatos, C.R., Kales, A. (1982) Psychotherapy with night-terror patients. *Am. J. Psychother.,* **36**, 399–407.

5   Allen, R.M. (1983) Attenuation of drug-induced anxiety dreams and pavor nocturnus by benzodiazepines. *J. Clin. Psychiatry,* **44**, 106–8.

6   Kales, A., Soldatos, C.R., Kales, J.D. (1987) Sleep disorders: insomnia, sleepwalking, night terrors, nightmares, and enuresis. *Ann. Intern. Med.,* **106**, S82–92.

7   Broughton, R.J. (1968) Sleep disorders: disorders of arousal? Enuresis, somnambulism, and nightmares occur in confusional states of arousal, not in 'dreaming sleep'. *Science,* **159**, 1070–8.

8   Kales, A., Soldatos, C.R., Bixler, E.O., Ladda, R.L., Charney, D.S., Weber, G. *et al.* (1980) Hereditary factors in sleepwalking and night terrors. *Br. J. Psychiatry,* **137**, 111–18.

9   Pradalier, A., Giroud, M., Dry, J. (1987) Somnambulism, migraine and propranolol. *Headache,* **27**, 143–5.

10 Barabas, G., Ferrari, M., Matthews, W.S. (1983) Childhood migraine and somnambulism. *Neurology,* **33**, 948–9.

11 Barabas, G., Matthews, W.S., Ferrari, M. (1984) Somnambulism in children with Tourette syndrome. *Dev. Med. Child Neurol.,* **26**, 457–60.

12 Kales, A., Soldatos, C.R., Caldwell, A.B., Kales, J.D., Humphrey, F.J., Charney, D.S. *et al.* (1980) Somnambulism. Clinical characteristics and personality patterns. *Arch. Gen. Psychiatry,* 37, 1406–10.

13 Klackenberg, G. (1982) Somnambulism in childhood – prevalence, course and behavioral correlations. A prospective longitudinal study (6–16 years). *Acta Paediatr. Scand.,* **71**, 495–9.

14 Hublin, C., Kaprio, J., Partinen, M., Heikkila, K., Koskenvuo, M. (1997) Prevalence and genetics of sleepwalking: a population-based twin study. *Neurology,* **48**, 177–81.

15 Oswald, I., Evans, J. (1985) On serious violence during sleep-walking. *Br. J. Psychiatry,* **147**, 688–91.

16 Rauch, P.K., Stern, T.A. (1986) Life-threatening injuries resulting from sleepwalking and night terrors. *Psychosomatics,* **27**, 62–4.

17 Broughton, R., Billings, R., Cartwright, R., Doucette, D., Edmeads, J., Edwardh, M. *et al.* (1994) Homicidal somnambulism: a case report. *Sleep,* **17**, 253–64.

18 Frank, N.C., Spirito, A., Stark, L., Owens-Stively, J. (1997) The use of scheduled awakenings to eliminate childhood sleepwalking. *J. Pediatr. Psychol.*, **22**, 345–53.

19 Schenck, C.H., Bundlie, S.R., Ettinger, M.G., Mahowald, M.W. (1986) Chronic behavioral disorders of human REM sleep: a new category of parasomnia. *Sleep*, **9**, 293–308.

20 Reese, N.B., Garcia-Rill, E., Skinner, R.D. (1995) The pedunculopontine nucleus – auditory input, arousal and pathophysiology. *Prog. Neurobiol.*, **47**, 105–33.

21 Schenck, C.H., Bundlie, S.R., Mahowald, M.W. (1996) Delayed emergence of a parkinsonian disorder in 38 per cent of 29 older men initially diagnosed with idiopathic rapid eye movement sleep behaviour disorder. *Neurology*, **46**, 388–93.

22 Schenck, C.H., Mahowald, M.W. (1996) Long-term, nightly benzodiazepine treatment of injurious parasomnias and other disorders of disrupted nocturnal sleep in 170 adults. *Am. J. Med.*, **100**, 333–7.

23 Schenck, C.H., Hurwitz, T.D., Mahowald, M.W. (1993) Symposium: normal and abnormal REM sleep regulation: REM sleep behaviour disorder: an update on a series of 96 patients and a review of the world literature. *J. Sleep Res.*, 2, 224–31.

24 Sforza, E., Krieger, J., Petiau, C. (1997) REM sleep behavior disorder: clinical and physiopathological findings. *Sleep Medicine Reviews,* **1**, 57–69.

25 Scheuler, W., Rappelsberger, P., Schmatz, F., Pastelak-Price, C., Petsche, H., Kubicki, S. (1990) Periodicity analysis of sleep EEG in the second and minute ranges – example of application in different alpha activities in sleep. *Electroencephalogr. Clin. Neurophysiol.*, **76**, 222–34.

26 Lavigne, G.J., Montplaisir, J.Y. (1994) Restless legs syndrome and sleep bruxism: prevalence and association among Canadians. *Sleep,* **17**, 739–43.

27 Ancoli-Israel, S., Kripke, D.F., Mason, W., Kaplan, O.J. (1985) Sleep apnea and periodic movements in an aging sample. *J. Gerontol.*, **40**, 419–25.

28 Hening, W., Allen, R., Earley, C., Kushida, C., Picchietti; D., Silber, M. (1999) The treatment of restless legs syndrome and periodic limb movement disorder. An American Academy of Sleep Medicine Review. *Sleep,* **22**, 970–99.

29 Hening, W., Allen, R., Earley, C., Kushida, C., Picchietti, D., Silber, M. (1999) The treatment of restless legs syndrome and periodic limb movement disorder. An American Academy of Sleep Medicine Review. *Sleep,* **22**, 970–99.

30 Chesson, A.L., Wise, M., Davila, D., Johnson, S., Littner, M., Anderson, W.M. *et al.* (1999) Practice parameters for the treatment of

restless legs syndrome and periodic limb movement disorder. An American Academy of Sleep Medicine Report. Standards of Practice Committee of the American Academy of Sleep Medicine. *Sleep,* **22,** 961–18.

31 Peled, R., Lavie, P. (1987) Double-blind evaluation of clonazepam on periodic leg movements in sleep. *J. Neurol. Neurosurg. Psychiatry,* **50,** 1679–81.

32 Earley, C.J., Connor, J.R., Beard, J.L., Malecki, E.A., Epstein, D.K., Allen, R.P. (2000) Abnormalities in CSF concentrations of ferritin and transferrin in restless legs syndrome. *Neurology,* **54,** 1698–700.

33 Davis, B.J., Rajput, A., Rajput, M.L., Aul, E.A., Eichhorn, G.R. (2000) A randomized, double-blind placebo-controlled trial of iron in restless legs syndrome. *Eur. Neurol.,* **43,** 70–5.

34 Benes, H., Kurella, B., Kummer, J., Kazenwadel, J., Selzer, R., Kohnen, R. (1999) Rapid onset of action of levodopa in restless legs syndrome: a double-blind, randomized, multicenter, crossover trial. *Sleep,* **22,** 1073–81.

35 Trenkwalder, C., Stiasny, K., Pollmacher, T., Wetter, T., Schwarz, J., Kohnen, R. *et al.* (1995) L-dopa therapy of uremic and idiopathic restless legs syndrome: a double-blind, crossover trial. *Sleep,* **18,** 681–8.

36 Wetter, T.C., Stiasny, K., Winkelmann, J., Buhlinger, A., Brandenburg, U., Penzel, T. *et al.* (1999) A randomized controlled study of pergolide in patients with restless legs syndrome. *Neurology,* **52,** 944–50.

37 Lugaresi, E., Cirignotta, F., Coccagna, G., Piana, C. (1980) Some epidemiological data on snoring and cardiocirculatory disturbances. *Sleep,* **3,** 221–4.

38 Norton, P.G., Dunn, E.V. (1985) Snoring as a risk factor for disease: an epidemiological survey. *BMJ,* **291,** 630–2.

39 Young, T., Palta, M., Dempsey, J., Skatrud, J., Weber, S., Badr, S. (1993) The occurrence of sleep-disordered breathing among middle-aged adults. *N. Engl. J. Med.,* **328,** 1230–5.

40 Ohayon, M.M., Guilleminault, C., Priest, R.G., Caulet, M. (1997) Snoring and breathing pauses during sleep: telephone interview survey of a United Kingdom population sample. *BMJ,* **314,** 860–3.

41 Bloom, J.W., Kaltenborn, W.T., Quan, S.F. (1988) Risk factors in a general population for snoring. Importance of cigarette smoking and obesity. *Chest,* **93,** 678–83.

42 Koskenvuo, M., Kaprio, J., Partinen, M., Langinvainio, H., Sarna, S., Heikkila, K. (1985) Snoring as a risk factor for hypertension and angina pectoris. *Lancet,* **1,** 893–6.

43 Koskenvuo, M., Kaprio, J., Telakivi, T., Partinen, M., Heikkila, K., Sarna, S. (1987) Snoring as a risk factor for ischaemic heart disease and stroke in men. *BMJ,* **294,** 16–19.

44 Palomaki, H., Partinen, M., Juvela, S., Kaste, M. (1989) Snoring as a risk factor for sleep-related brain infarction. *Stroke,* **20** 1311–15.

45 Stradling, J.R., Negus, T.W., Smith, D., Langford, B. (1998) Mandibular advancement devices for the control of snoring. *Eur Respir. J.,* **11**, 447–50.

46 Bloch, K.E., Iseli, A., Zhang, J.N., Xie, X., Kaplan, V., Stoeckli, P.W. *et al.* (2000) A randomized, controlled crossover trial of two oral appliances for sleep apnea treatment. *Am. J. Respir. Crit. Care Med.,* **162**, 246–51.

47 Schmidt-Nowara, W., Lowe, A., Wiegand, L., Cartwright, R., Perez-Guerra, F., Menn, S. (1995) Oral appliances for the treatment of snoring and obstructive sleep apnea: a review. *Sleep,* **18**, 501–10.

48 Series, F., St Pierre, S., Carrier, G. (1992) Effects of surgical correction of nasal obstruction in the treatment of obstructive sleep apnea. *Am. Rev. Respir. Dis.,* **146**, 1261–5.

49 Mortimore, I.L., Bradley, P.A., Murray, J.A., Douglas, N.J. (1996) Uvulopalatopharyngoplasty may compromise nasal CPAP therapy in sleep apnea syndrome. *Am. J. Respir. Crit. Care Med.,* **154**, 1759–62.

50 Hoffstein, V., Mateika, S., Nash, S. (1996) Comparing perceptions and measurements of snoring. *Sleep,* **19**, 783–9.

51 Powell, N.B., Riley, R.W., Troell, R.J., Li, K., Blumen, M.B., Guilleminault, C. (1998) Radiofrequency volumetric tissue reduction of the palate in subjects with sleep-disordered breathing. *Chest,* **113**, 1163–74.

52 Boudewyns, A., Van De, H.P. (2000) Temperature-controlled radiofrequency tissue volume reduction of the soft palate (somnoplasty) in the treatment of habitual snoring: results of a European multicenter trial. *Acta Otolaryngol.,* **120**, 981–5.

53 Emery, B.E., Flexon, P.B. (2000) Radiofrequency volumetric tissue reduction of the soft palate: a new treatment for snoring. *Laryngoscope,* **110**, 1092–8.

54 Li, K.K., Powell, N.B., Riley, R.W., Troell, R.J., Guilleminault, C. (2000) Radiofrequency volumetric reduction of the palate: An extended follow-up study. *Otolaryngol. Head Neck Surg.,* **122**, 410–14.

55 Mellins, R.B., Balfour, H.H., Turino, G.M., Winters, R.W. (1970) Failure of automatic control of ventilation (Ondines curse). Report of an infant born with this syndrome and review of the literature. *Medicine,* **49**, 487–504.

56 Xie, A., Rutherford, R., Rankin, F., Wong, B., Bradley, T.D. (1995) Hypocapnia and increased ventilatory responsiveness in patients with idiopathic central sleep apnea. *Am J. Respir. Crit. Care Med.,* **152**, 1950–5.

57 Guilleminault, C., van den Hoed, J., Mitler, M.M. (1978) Clinical

overview of the sleep apnea syndromes, in C. Guilleminault, W.C. Dement (eds). *Sleep Apnea Syndromes,* pp. 1–12. New York: Liss.

58 White, D.P., Zwillich, C.W., Pickett, C.K., Douglas, N.J., Findley, L.J., Weil, J.V (1982) Central sleep apnea. Improvement with acetazolamide therapy. *Arch. Intern. Med.,* **142,** 1816–19.

59 Bradley, T.D., McNicholas, W.T., Rutherford, R., Popkin, J., Zamel, N., Phillipson, E.A. (1986) Clinical and physiologic heterogeneity of the central sleep apnea syndrome. *Am. Rev. Respir. Dis.,* **134,** 217–21.

60 American Sleep Disorders Association. (1999) Sleep-related breathing disorders in adults: recommendations for syndrome definition and measurement techniques in clinical research. The Report of an American Academy of Sleep Medicine Task Force. *Sleep,* **22,** 667–89.

61 Issa, F.G., Sullivan, C.E. (1986) Reversal of central sleep apnea using nasal CPAP. *Chest,* **90,** 165–71.

62 Hoffstein, V., Slutsky, A.S. (1987) Central sleep apnea reversed by continuous positive airway pressure. *Am. Rev. Respir. Dis.,* **135,** 1210–12.

63 McNicholas, W.T., Carter, J.L., Rutherford, R., Zamel, N., Phillipson, E.A. (1982) Beneficial effect of oxygen in primary alveolar hypoventilation with central sleep apnea. *Am. Rev. Respir. Dis.,* **125,** 773–5.

64 Bader, G., Lavigne, G. (2000) Sleep bruxism; an overview of an oromandibular sleep movement disorder. *Sleep Medicine Reviews,* **4,** 27–43.

65 Jarvelin, M.R., Moilanen, I., Kangas, P., Moring, K., Vikevainen-Tervonen, L., Huttunen, N.P. *et al.* (1991) Aetiological and precipitating factors for childhood enuresis. *Acta Paediatr. Scand.,* **80,** 361–9.

66 Maizels, M., Rosenbaum, D. (1985) Successful treatment of nocturnal enuresis: a practical approach. *Prim. Care,* **12,** 621–35.

67 Moilanen, I., Tirkkonen, T., Jarvelin, M.R., Linna, S.L., Almqvist, F., Piha, J. *et al.* (1998) A follow-up of enuresis from childhood to adolescence. *Br. J. Urol.,* **81** (Suppl. 3), 94–7.

Breathing during sleep in patients with COPD

Patients with chronic obstructive pulmonary disease (COPD) become more hypoxaemic during sleep than when awake, even more hypoxaemic than during exercise.[1] They become slightly more hypoxaemic as they fall into non-REM sleep, and much more hypoxaemic in REM sleep when oxygen saturation may fall to extremely low levels,[2] especially in those whose oxygenation is poor even before sleep (Figure 9.1). This sleep-related hypoxaemia affects the cardiovascular and haematological systems and is thus of clinical significance. This chapter will discuss the pathogenesis, complications and therapy of this phenomenon.

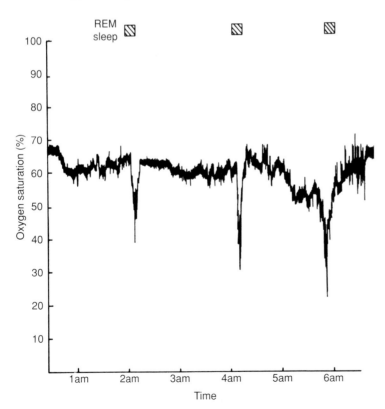

Figure 9.1
Overnight oxygen saturation in a patient with chronic obstructive pulmonary disease (COPD) showing marked desaturation in REM sleep.

Aetiology

HYPOVENTILATION

The drop in oxygenation occurs despite continuing ventilation – this is not a sleep apnoea phenomenon, at least in the vast majority of COPD patients. The mild desaturation in non-REM sleep seems largely to be due to the slight fall in minute ventilation in non-REM found in both normal subjects[3] and in patients with COPD.[4,5] During REM sleep there is a marked fall in ventilation in normal subjects with rapid shallow breathing leading to much lower alveolar ventilation.[3] The hypoventilation is most marked during periods of REM sleep in which there are frequent eye movements – so-called phasic REM sleep.[6] Patients with COPD also hypoventilate in REM sleep[7] (Figure 9.2). Breathing patterns during REM sleep are similar in patients with COPD and normal subjects.[8] Recent studies in COPD patients suggest that the decrease in minute ventilation from wakefulness to REM sleep is of the order of 32 per cent.[9] The rapid shallow breathing when combined with the greater physiological deadspace in patients with COPD, will give rise to a larger drop in alveolar ventilation during REM in COPD, so contributing to the pronounced desaturation. It is possible that this fall in ventilation may account for all of the hypoxaemia found during REM sleep in COPD,[10] but this thesis has not been tested.

Many factors contribute to the hypoventilation during sleep in COPD. In non-REM sleep, normal subjects hypoventilate despite an increase in the drive to breathing as assessed by the mouth occlusion pressure.[11] The ventilatory response to increased resistance is impaired during sleep[12] which combined with the increase in upper airways resistance during non-REM sleep[13] contributes to the drop in ventilation. The decrease in basal metabolic rate

Figure 9.2
Tidal volume (V_T), oxygen saturation % (SaO_2) and sleep stage in a patient with COPD illustrating the drop in oxygen saturation and the irregular hypoventilation in REM sleep. (Adapted from Fletcher,[7] with permission.)

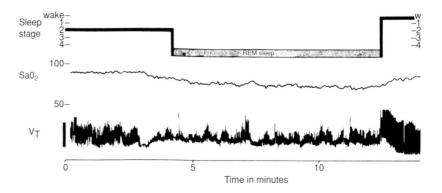

during sleep[14] may also contribute to the hypoventilation which is permitted by falls in the ventilatory responses to hypoxia[15] and hypercapnia.[16]

The marked further falls in oxygenation during REM sleep are not due to further rises in upper airways resistance which seems to be lower in REM sleep than in non-REM sleep.[13] Instead the mechanism seems to be alteration of central respiratory control which generates the irregular pattern of breathing characteristic of REM sleep. The very shallow breathing found during periods of dense eye movements in normal subjects' sleep[6] (*see* Figure 1.8) also occurs in patients with COPD[17] (Figure 9.3). In addition, during REM sleep there is hypotonicity of the postural muscles and thus the intercostal muscles' contribution to ventilation falls, leaving the diaphragm with a larger role.[18] However, patients with COPD have low flat and inefficient diaphragms and so this diminishes ventilation further. The ventilatory responses to both hypoxia[15] and hypercapnia[16] are reduced in REM sleep to about a third of normal thus reducing the body's normal defence mechanism to such hypoventilation.

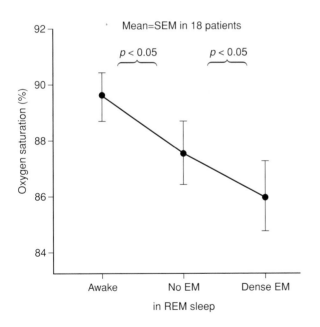

Figure 9.3
Oxygen saturation during wakefullness and rapid eye movement (REM) sleep divided into periods of REM sleep with no or dense eye movements (EM). (Adapted from George,[17] with permission.)

OTHER MECHANISMS

Early reports that lung volume fell during REM sleep in patients with COPD[4] have not been substantiated by a subsequent and technically superior study.[5] Similarly, there is no good evidence that increased mismatching occurs as a primary event during sleep to contribute to the hypoxaemia,[19] although ventilation/perfusion matching is bound to be secondarily affected by the hypoventilation.

COPD COMBINED WITH OSAHS

Both COPD and obstructive sleep apnoea/hypopnoea syndrome (OSAHS) are common conditions, and by chance they will co-exist in occasional patients. Indeed, the limited data available suggest that the frequency of OSAHS in patients with COPD is similar to that in the general population at around two per cent.[20] Studies in patients with OSAHS suggest that about 10 per cent of them have some degree of COPD.[21] Patients with both COPD and OSAHS have 'broad band' oxygen desaturation during sleep (*see* Figure 2.16), not the typical narrow REM desaturation found in simple COPD (*see* Figure 9.1).

Consequences of sleep hypoxaemia in COPD

Pulmonary hypertension, polycythaemia and impaired sleep are the best documented potential sequelae of nocturnal hypoxaemia in COPD.

PULMONARY HYPERTENSION

Pulmonary arterial pressure rises as oxygen saturation falls during sleep[22] with an average rise of 1 mm Hg in mean pulmonary arterial pressure for every one per cent fall in oxygen saturation. The clinical significance of these rises is not known. However, both logic and experimental animal data[23] suggest that such rises occurring many times per night for years or even decades are likely to have deleterious cardiovascular consequences and contribute to the development of cor pulmonale.

POLYCYTHAEMIA

Both animal experiments[23] and measurements in patients with COPD[24] suggest that nocturnal hypoxaemia may contribute to the development of secondary polycythaemia. However, it appears that marked hypoxaemia with oxygen saturation falling below 60 per cent is required before there are measurable rises in serum erythropoetin levels.[24]

SLEEP QUALITY

Patients with COPD sleep poorly according to both subjective[25] and objective[26] reports. However, there is no evidence as yet that this has deleterious effects on their daytime sleepiness.[27]

OTHER EFFECTS

Patients with COPD have more ventricular dysrhythmias during sleep than normal subjects, but there is no evidence that these are harmful. Also, patients with COPD die more often at night than during the day, but it is unclear whether this relates to sleep in any way.

CONSEQUENCES OF COPD COMBINED WITH OSAHS

Patients with both conditions are at increased risk of pulmonary hypertension,[28] right heart failure[29] and carbon dioxide retention.[30] This is presumably because they have two causes of nocturnal hypoventilation, which is thus more severe than in patients with COPD alone.

Role of studies of breathing and oxygenation during sleep

Routine sleep studies have been suggested in patients with COPD for four reasons:

- To identify patients with both COPD and OSAHS.
- To identify patients who are excessive desaturators.
- To select patients who would benefit from nocturnal oxygen therapy.
- To guide the oxygen concentration used.

The rationale for these indications is examined below. There seems to be no clinical value in performing sleep studies to detect OSAHS in all patients with COPD as patients with COPD and OSAHS appear to have the typical symptoms of OSAHS[20,21] and these should be the trigger for a sleep study.

Patients who are most hypoxaemic when awake become the most hypoxaemic during sleep. Indeed, sleeping oxygenation can be predicted from awake oxygenation, arterial PCO_2 and REM sleep duration,[20] but there is a large residual variance (Figure 9.4). To try to establish whether this variance was clinically significant, survival was compared in those who became less

Figure 9.4
Relationship between oxygenation when awake and the lowest oxygen saturation (S_aO_2) during sleep in 97 patients with COPD. (Adapted from Connaughton,[20] with permission.)

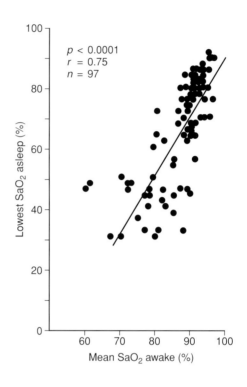

Figure 9.5
Survival curves for patients who were more hypoxaemic at night than predicted from their awake oxygen saturation and CO_2 level in comparison to those who were less hypoxaemic than predicted. There was no difference in survival between the two groups. (Adapted from Connaughton,[20] with permission.)

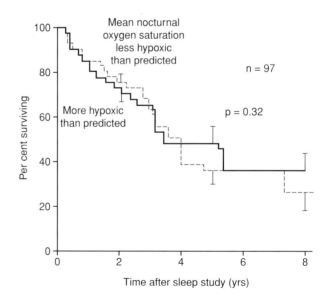

hypoxaemic during sleep than predicted from the waking oxygenation with survival in those who became more hypoxaemic than predicted. This analysis[20] showed no difference in survival (Figure 9.5) and so there appears to be no be value in identifying excess desaturators and no value in performing routine sleep studies in patients with COPD.

Treatment of nocturnal hypoxaemia

OXYGEN

Unsurprisingly, nocturnal oxygen therapy increases oxygenation during sleep in patients with COPD.[2] Nocturnal oxygen therapy also improves survival in hypoxaemic patients with COPD.[31,32] Both the MRC[31] and Nocturnal Oxygen Therapy[32] trials used daytime oxygenation to select patients for nocturnal oxygen therapy. There are no data indicating that measurement of nocturnal oxygenation can usefully contribute to the selection of patients for nocturnal oxygen therapy, indeed the available data suggests it does not.[33-35] Chaouat[35] studied 76 patients with daytime arterial oxygen tensions of 56–69 mm Hg who spent more than 30 per cent of the night with oxygen saturations of less than 90 per cent. They were randomized to nocturnal air or oxygen therapy designed to keep saturation above 90 per cent, but there was no difference in survival or pulmonary arterial pressure after two years.

There is no evidence that sleep studies should be performed with the patient receiving supplemental oxygen therapy in order to assess the optimal concentration of oxygen to provide at night. Thus, although nocturnal oxygen therapy is the treatment of choice for sleep-related hypoxaemia in patients with COPD, there is no evidence that sleep studies help with the selection of which patients should receive nocturnal oxygen or with the choice of oxygen concentration to use.

NIPPV

Nasal intermittent positive pressure ventilation (NIPPV) can improve both nocturnal oxygenation and nocturnal CO_2 levels. Some patients prefer NIPPV to oxygen therapy[36,37] and it is also a safer alternative for those who smoke. Nevertheless, NIPPV on its own does not have as great an effect on oxygenation as oxygen therapy,[38] whereas the combination of NIPPV and oxygen has a greater effect on both day and sleeping arterial blood gas tensions as well as on sleep pattern and quality of life.[39] Many patients with COPD will not tolerate NIPPV, and certainly COPD patients are much more difficult to both start and keep on NIPPV than patients with neuro-muscular or chest wall disease.[37] There is a need for large clinical trials of the effect of NIPPV on survival in hypoxaemic patients with COPD.

MEDICATIONS

Respiratory stimulants tried include almitrine,[40] medroxyprogesterone acetate, acetazolamide and theophylline, but none have established a significant role in clinical practice. The same applies to bronchodilators and to REM sleep suppressants, such as protriptyline, whose utility is limited by anticholinergic side-effects.[41]

TREATMENT OF COPD COMBINED WITH OSAHS

When these two conditions co-exist, therapy of the OSAHS appears to be critical.[42] Indeed, those patients in whom nocturnal oxygen therapy was

Figure 9.6
Arterial oxygen and carbon dioxide tensions in mm Hg in patients with both COPD and OSAHS at baseline and following treatment for OSAHS (open symbols) or treatment for COPD alone (closed symbols). The p values indicate significant improvements in arterial blood gas tensions with treatment of the OSAHS component. (Adapted from Fletcher,42 with permission.)

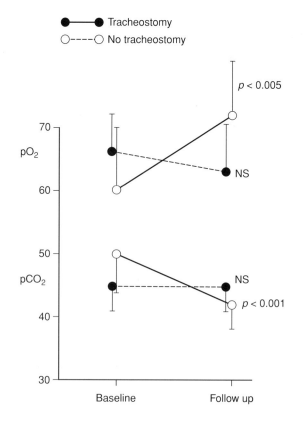

given deteriorated, whereas those in whom the OSAHS was treated (Figure 9.6) showed improvements in arterial blood gas tensions and pulmonary haemodynamics.[42]

Conclusion

Patients with COPD become hypoxaemic during REM sleep due to hypoventilation. This is a normal sleep-related physiological change that has pathophysiological consequences by contributing to polycythaemia, pulmonary hypertension and sleep disturbance. There is no role for sleep studies unless co-existing OSAHS is suspected on history. Nocturnal oxygen is the current treatment of choice, although the role of NIPPV may increase.

References

1 Mulloy, E., McNicholas, W.T. (1996) Ventilation and gas exchange during sleep and exercise in severe COPD. *Chest*, **109**, 387–94.

2 Douglas, N.J., Calverley, P.M., Leggett, R.J., Brash, H.M., Flenley, D.C., Brezinova, V. (1979) Transient hypoxaemia during sleep in chronic bronchitis and emphysema. *Lancet*, **1**, 1–4.

3 Douglas, N.J., White, D.P., Pickett, C.K., Weil, J.V., Zwillich, C.W. (1982) Respiration during sleep in normal man. *Thorax*, **37**, 840–4.

4 Hudgel, D.W., Martin, R.J., Capehart, M., Johnson, B., Hill, P. (1983) Contribution of hypoventilation to sleep oxygen desaturation in chronic obstructive pulmonary disease. *J. Appl. Physiol.*, **55**, 669–77.

5 Ballard, R.D., Clover, C.W., Suh, B.Y. (1995) Influence of sleep on respiratory function in emphysema. *Am. J. Respir. Crit. Care Med.*, **151**, 945–51.

6 Gould, G.A., Gugger, M., Molloy, J., Tsara, V., Shapiro, C.M., Douglas, N.J. (1988) Breathing pattern and eye movement density during REM sleep in humans. *Am. Rev. Respir. Dis.*, **138**, 874–7.

7 Fletcher, E.C., Gray, B.A., Levin, D.C. (1983) Nonapneic mechanisms of arterial oxygen desaturation during rapid-eye-movement sleep. *J. Appl. Physiol.*, **54**, 632–9.

8 Catterall, J.R., Calverley, P.M., Shapiro, C.M., Flenley, D.C., Douglas, N.J. (1985) Breathing and oxygenation during sleep are similar in normal men and normal women. *Am. Rev. Respir. Dis.*, **132**, 86–8.

9 Becker, H.F., Piper, A.J., Flynn, W.E., McNamara, S.G., Grunstein, R.R., Peter, J.H. *et al.* (1999) Breathing during sleep in patients with nocturnal desaturation. *Am. J. Respir. Crit. Care Med.*, **159**, 112–18.

10 Catterall, J.R., Calverley, P.M., MacNee, W., Warren, P.M., Shapiro, C.M., Douglas, N.J. *et al.* (1985) Mechanism of transient nocturnal hypoxemia in hypoxic chronic bronchitis and emphysema. *J. Appl. Physiol.*, **59**, 1698–703.

11 White, D.P. (1986) Occlusion pressure and ventilation during sleep in normal humans. *J. Appl. Physiol.*, **61**, 1279–87.

12 Wiegand, L., Zwillich, C.W., White, D.P. (1988) Sleep and the ventilatory response to resistive loading in normal men. *J. Appl. Physiol.*, **64**, 1186–95.

13 Hudgel, D.W., Martin, R.J., Johnson, B., Hill, P. (1984) Mechanics of the respiratory system and breathing pattern during sleep in normal humans. *J. Appl. Physiol.*, **56**, 133–7.

14 White, D.P., Weil, J.V., Zwillich, C.W. (1985) Metabolic rate and breathing during sleep. *J. Appl. Physiol.*, **59**, 384–91.

15 Douglas, N.J., White, D.P., Weil, J.V., Pickett, C.K., Martin, R.J., Hudgel, D.W. *et al.* (1982) Hypoxic ventilatory response decreases during sleep in normal men. *Am. Rev. Respir. Dis.*, 125, 286–9.

16 Douglas, N.J., White, D.P., Weil, J.V., Pickett, C.K., Zwillich, C.W. (1982) Hypercapnic ventilatory response in sleeping adults. *Am. Rev. Respir. Dis.*, **126**, 758–62.

17 George, C.F., West, P., Kryger, M.H. (1987) Oxygenation and breathing pattern during phasic and tonic REM in patients with chronic obstructive pulmonary disease. *Sleep*, **10**, 234–43.

18 White, J.E., Drinnan, M.J., Smithson, A.J., Griffiths, C.J., Gibson, G.J. (1995) Respiratory muscle activity during rapid eye movement (REM) sleep in patients with chronic obstructive pulmonary disease. *Thorax*, **50**, 376–82.

19 Catterall, J.R., Calverley, P.M., MacNee, W., Warren, P.M., Shapiro, C.M., Douglas, N.J. *et al.* (1985) Mechanism of transient nocturnal hypoxemia in hypoxic chronic bronchitis and emphysema. *J. Appl. Physiol.*, **59**, 1698–703.

20 Connaughton, J.J., Catterall, J.R., Elton, R.A., Stradling, J.R., Douglas, N.J. (1988) Do sleep studies contribute to the management of patients with severe chronic obstructive pulmonary disease? *Am. Rev. Respir. Dis.*, **138**, 341–4.

21 Chaouat, A., Weitzenblum, E., Krieger, J., Ifoundza, T., Oswald, M., Kessler, R. (1995) Association of chronic obstructive pulmonary disease and sleep apnea syndrome. *Am. J. Respir. Crit. Care Med.*, **151**, 82–6.

22 Boysen, P.G., Block, A.J., Wynne, J.W., Hunt, L.A., Flick, M.R. (1979) Nocturnal pulmonary hypertension in patients with chronic obstructive pulmonary disease. *Chest*, **76**, 536–42.

23 Moore-Gillon, J.C., Cameron, I.R. (1985) Right ventricular hyper-

trophy and polycythaemia in rats after intermittent exposure to hypoxia. *Clin. Sci. (Colch)*, **69**, 595–9.

24 Fitzpatrick, M.F., Mackay, T., Whyte, K.F., Allen, M., Tam, R.C., Dore, C.J. *et al.* (1993) Nocturnal desaturation and serum erythropoietin: a study in patients with chronic obstructive pulmonary disease and in normal subjects. *Clin. Sci. (Colch)*, **84**, 319–24.

25 Cormick, W., Olson, L.G., Hensley, M.J., Saunders, N.A. (1986) Nocturnal hypoxaemia and quality of sleep in patients with chronic obstructive lung disease. *Thorax*, **41**, 846–54.

26 Fleetham, J., West, P., Mezon, B., Conway, W., Roth, T., Kryger, M. (1982) Sleep, arousals, and oxygen desaturation in chronic obstructive pulmonary disease. The effect of oxygen therapy. *Am. Rev. Respir. Dis.*, **126**, 429–33.

27 Orr, W.C., Shamma-Othman, Z., Levin, D., Othman, J., Rundell, O.H. (1990) Persistent hypoxemia and excessive daytime sleepiness in chronic obstructive pulmonary disease (COPD). *Chest*, **97**, 583–5.

28 Weitzenblum, E., Krieger, J., Apprill, M., Vallee, E., Ehrhart, M., Ratomaharo, J. *et al.* (1988) Daytime pulmonary hypertension in patients with obstructive sleep apnea syndrome. *Am. Rev. Respir. Dis.*, **138**, 345–9.

29 Bradley, T.D., Rutherford, R., Grossman, R.F., Lue, F., Zamel, N., Moldofsky, H. *et al.* (1985) Role of daytime hypoxemia in the pathogenesis of right heart failure in the obstructive sleep apnea syndrome. *Am. Rev. Respir. Dis.*, **131**, 835–9.

30 Bradley, T.D., Rutherford, R., Lue, F., Moldofsky, H., Grossman, R.F., Zamel, N. *et al.* (1986) Role of diffuse airway obstruction in the hypercapnia of obstructive sleep apnea. *Am. Rev. Respir. Dis.*, **134**, 920–4.

31 Medical Research Council Working Party. (1981) Long term domiciliary oxygen therapy in chronic hypoxic cor pulmonale complicating chronic bronchitis and emphysema. *Lancet*, **1**, 681–6.

32 Nocturnal Oxygen Therapy Trial Group. (1980) Continuous or nocturnal oxygen therapy in hypoxemic chronic obstructive lung disease: a clinical trial. *Ann. Intern. Med.*, **93**, 391–8.

33 Fletcher, E.C., Luckett, R.A., Goodnight-White, S., Miller, C.C., Qian, W., Costarangos-Galarza, C. (1992) A double-blind trial of nocturnal supplemental oxygen for sleep desaturation in patients with chronic obstructive pulmonary disease and a daytime PaO_2 above 60 mm Hg. *Am. Rev. Respir. Dis.*, **145**, 1070–6.

34 Fletcher, E.C., Donner, C.F., Midgren, B., Zielinski, J., Levi-Valensi, P., Braghiroli, A. *et al.* (1992) Survival in COPD patients with a daytime PaO_2 greater than 60 mm Hg with and without nocturnal oxyhemoglobin desaturation. *Chest*, **101**, 649–55.

35 Chaouat, A., Weitzenblum, E., Kessler, R., Charpentier, C., Enrhart, M., Schott, R. *et al.* (1999) A randomized trial of nocturnal oxygen therapy in chronic obstructive pulmonary disease patients. *Eur. Respir. J.*, **14**, 1002–8.

36 Elliott, M.W., Simonds, A.K., Carroll, M.P., Wedzicha, J.A., Branthwaite, M.A. (1992) Domiciliary nocturnal nasal intermittent positive pressure ventilation in hypercapnic respiratory failure due to chronic obstructive lung disease: effects on sleep and quality of life. *Thorax*, **47**, 342–8.

37 Simonds, A.K., Elliott, M.W. (1995) Outcome of domiciliary nasal intermittent positive pressure ventilation in restrictive and obstructive disorders. *Thorax*, **50**, 604–9.

38 Lin, C.C. (1996) Comparison between nocturnal nasal positive pressure ventilation combined with oxygen therapy and oxygen monotherapy in patients with severe COPD. *Am. J. Respir. Crit. Care Med.*, **154**, 353–8.

39 Meecham Jones, D.J., Paul, E.A., Jones, P.W., Wedzicha, J.A. (1995) Nasal pressure support ventilation plus oxygen compared with oxygen therapy alone in hypercapnic COPD. *Am. J. Respir. Crit. Care Med.*, **152**, 538–44.

40 Connaughton, J.J., Douglas, N.J., Morgan, A.D., Shapiro, C.M., Critchley, J.A., Pauly, N. *et al.* (1985) Almitrine improves oxygenation when both awake and asleep in patients with hypoxia and carbon dioxide retention caused by chronic bronchitis and emphysema. *Am. Rev. Respir. Dis.*, **132**, 206–10.

41 Series, F., Marc, I., Cormier, Y., La Forge, J. (1993) Long-term effects of protriptyline in patients with chronic obstructive pulmonary disease. *Am. Rev. Respir. Dis.*, **147**, 1487–90.

42 Fletcher, E.C., Schaaf, J.W., Miller, J., Fletcher, J.G. (1987) Long-term cardiopulmonary sequelae in patients with sleep apnea and chronic lung disease. *Am. Rev. Respir. Dis.*, **135**, 525–33.

Nocturnal asthma

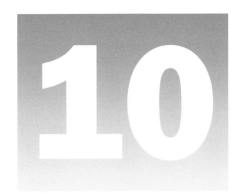

Introduction

Asthma is common, occurring in approximately five per cent of the population at some time in their lives, and the frequency is reportedly rising. Many people with asthma are troubled from time to time by nocturnal cough, wheeze or breathlessness and in some these sleep-related symptoms are the most troublesome aspects of their asthma. It must be stressed at the outset that nocturnal asthma is not a different condition from asthma, merely one manifestation of the disease, and one that tends to mainly affect those with more severe asthma.

Recognition of nocturnal asthma is not new. In 1698, Dr (later Sir) John Floyer wrote[1] about his own asthma:

> I have observed the fit always to happen after sleep in the night, when the nerves are filled with windy spirits . . . the diaphragm seems stiff and tied . . . it is not without much difficulty moved downwards.

Floyer was not only well in advance of the medical profession in recognizing the phenomenon and its link with sleep, but he also correctly identified the importance of the nervous system although twenty-first century neurophysiological explanations are more refined!

Epidemiology

Nocturnal asthma, defined as the intermittent presence of nocturnal cough, wheeze or breathlessness sufficient to interfere with sleep, is extremely common among asthma sufferers. Seventy-five per cent of asthmatic subjects referred to a hospital clinic had nocturnal symptoms,[2] whereas among those attending family practitioners 73 per cent had nocturnal symptoms at least once a week and 39 per cent nightly.[3] A population survey found that more than 85 per cent of asthmatic subjects woke from time to time, and 30 per cent woke more than 20 times a year with nocturnal symptoms.[4] The new development of nocturnal symptoms is often the warning sign patients use to identify deterioration in their asthmatic control and the need for intensification of therapy. In patients admitted to hospital with attacks of asthma most will report recent nocturnal problems.

When nocturnal asthma has been defined – in my opinion wrongly – by expiratory flow rates **irrespective of symptoms**, two-thirds of asthma sufferers have their lowest peak flows of the 24 hours during the period 10 pm to 8 am with a mean amplitude of variation of peak flow rate of 29 per cent.[5] Thus, overnight bronchial narrowing is common in asthmatics.

Mechanism and timing of nocturnal airway narrowing

If a sufficiently sensitive test is used, normal subjects can also be shown to have overnight airway narrowing.[6] However, this narrowing is trivial and insufficient to cause any symptoms. In the largest comparative series, the mean overnight fall in peak expiratory flow rate in normal subjects was eight per cent, whereas that in subjects with asthma was 50 per cent.[7] Nevertheless, the changes in normal subjects are synchronous with the much larger variations in asthmatics, suggesting a common mechanism. In other words, the bronchial narrowing overnight in asthma is an exaggeration of a normal physiological response in the same way that asthma sufferers have an increased airway narrowing response to a wide variety of other factors which may produce mild airway narrowing in normal subjects, such as methacholine and cold air.

Thus, nocturnal bronchial narrowing appears to be a circadian phenomenon. This is further supported by the observation that the timing of sleep in shiftworking asthmatics determines the timing of the 'overnight' bronchoconstriction[8,9] with rapid changes in the times of airway narrowing at the time of sleeping changes. The central role of sleep is further reinforced by a study showing that if asthmatic subjects are kept awake all night the magnitude of the overnight fall in peak flow rate is greatly reduced.[10] These data thus suggest that sleep time plays a major role in controlling overnight airway narrowing. However, many other possible causes for overnight bronchoconstriction have been proposed and these will be briefly reviewed.

Allergens in bedding are not the generic cause for nocturnal asthma as non-allergic asthmatic sufferers are just as likely to have nocturnal problems.[5] However, exposure to allergens can increase bronchial reactivity in predisposed subjects[11] and increased bronchial reactivity results in worsening of nocturnal asthma[12] (Figure 10.1). Thus, scrupulous exclusion of house

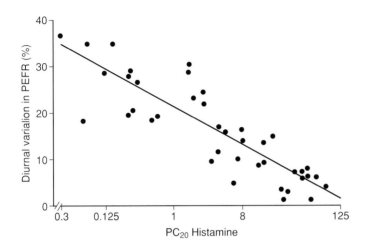

Figure 10.1
Relationship between diurnal variation in peak flow and bronchial reactivity to histamine showing the more twitchy the airway the greater the diurnal variation in peak flow. (Adapted from Ryan (1982) Bronchial responsiveness to histamine relationship to diurnal variation of peak flow rate, improvement after bronchodilator, and airway calibre. *Thorax*, 37, 423–9 with permission from BMJ Publishing Group.) PC_{20} is the concentration of inhaled histamine causing a 20 per cent fall in the FEV_1.

dust mite from the bedroom can decrease nocturnal asthma[13,14] by decreasing airway twitchiness rather than by having a direct effect on allergen-induced immediate-type bronchoconstriction. However, strict allergen avoidance is difficult to achieve in routine clinical practice.[15]

It has been suggested that airway cooling either due to decreased core body temperature or to the tendency for bedrooms to be cool at night might be a cause, as airway cooling is a potent cause of airway narrowing in asthmatic subjects. However, nocturnal asthma occurs despite a constant temperature over the 24 hours[16] so this seems an unlikely explanation. Similarly, lying down in bed seems an improbable explanation as asthmas left lying for 24 hours still exhibit overnight airway narrowing[17] and lying down does not produce sustained bronchoconstriction.[18]

Gastro-oesophageal reflux (GER) is common in asthmatics and has been implicated in nocturnal attacks. There is some evidence that in patients with severe GER, episodes of reflux are associated in time with increases in airflow resistance[19] but this is disputed[20] and there is no convincing evidence of a cause and effect relationship for asthmatic subjects in general.[21,22] Further, there is conflicting evidence whether treating GER benefits nocturnal asthma.[23,24] A systematic review concluded there is no clear evidence to support GER treatment with the aim of improving nocturnal or diurnal asthma.[25] Thus the link between GER and nocturnal asthma remains unproven.

Bronchial hyper-reactivity shows significant circadian variation with greatest sensitivity at night to a wide variety of stimuli, including inhaled histamine, allergens and cAMP.[26,27] However, because the airways are narrower at night, the greater reactivity could merely reflect differences in airway calibre prior to inhalation. The suggestion that this could be a normal physiological response is supported by evidence that bronchoconstriction to methacholine is increased in the morning in normal subjects.[28] Nevertheless, there is an increased reactivity to skin prick tests in the evening, although this is markedly reduced in the morning,[29] so there may be a genuine circadian element to hyper-reactivity.

A few asthmatics who are heavy snorers or have full-blown obstructive sleep apnoea/hypopnoea syndrome (OSAHS) seem to narrow their airways at night as a consequence of their snoring.[30] It is not clear how common this phenomenon is, but in my experience it is unusual.

Effector mechanisms producing nocturnal airway narrowing

Overnight bronchial narrowing is due to a circadian variation synchronized by sleep time. The possible mechanism producing the narrowing include the following.

INCREASED PARASYMPATHETIC TONE

Parasympathetic tone increases during sleep.[31] Cholinergic blockade studies suggest that much, but not all, of overnight bronchial narrowing is due to an overnight increase in parasympathetic tone.[32,33] Recent circadian desynchronization studies have confirmed that increased vagal tone may be a major cause of nocturnal bronchoconstriction.[34]

DECREASED NON-ADRENERGIC NON-CHOLINERGIC BRONCHODILATING TONE

The non-adrenergic non-cholinergic (NANC) nervous system produces bronchodilation in man. The activity of the airway NANC system has been shown to be impaired in the early morning[35,36] and this would contribute to bronchoconstriction then.

Thus, sleep-related changes in neural tone contribute to nocturnal asthma. However, as overnight bronchoconstriction may occur in transplanted lungs which have been denervated[37] this is not the only mechanism.

CIRCADIAN CHANGES IN CIRCULATING HORMONES

Both circulating cortisol and catechol levels fall overnight and it has been suggested that they may contribute to the development of nocturnal asthma.

However, synchrony does not prove causation and neither infusion of hydrocortisone[17] nor of catechols[38] prevents nocturnal airway narrowing. Further, nocturnal asthma may prove remarkably resistant to high-dose oral steroids in some patients.

AIRWAY INFLAMMATORY CHANGES

Despite considerable recent interest, there is conflicting evidence whether there are consistent changes in airway inflammatory cell populations or mediators in nocturnal asthma.[39–46] Increased inflammatory cells in bronchoalveolar lavage specimens at 0400 hours have been found in some,[41,42] but not all[39,47] studies. Bronchial biopsies at 0400 hours showed no change in cell populations.[41,45] Further, there is no evidence of any causal relationship between changes in inflammatory cell numbers and nocturnal airway narrowing.[41,45,47] One study has suggested a correlation between the FEV_1 at 0400 hours and CD4+ cells in alveolar tissue[40] but no causative role has been established. Increases in bronchoalveolar lavage cytokines eosinophil cationic protein[41] and IL1-beta[46] have been found in some studies. There is no evidence of increase expression of vascular adhesion molecules in at 0400 hours in patients with nocturnal asthma.[43] Thus, this confusing situation could be summarized by stating some inconsistent changes in inflammatory markers have been found overnight in the lungs of patients with nocturnal asthma, but their relevance is not yet clear. Indeed, so many variables have been studied that some were likely to be positive merely by chance alone.

EFFECTOR MECHANISMS – CONCLUSIONS

The circadian rhythm of airway calibre seems to be synchronized by sleep and to be largely neurally effected through increased cholinergic bronchoconstrictor and decreased non-adrenergic non-cholinergic bronchodilator tone overnight, but other factors may play a role (Figure 10.2).

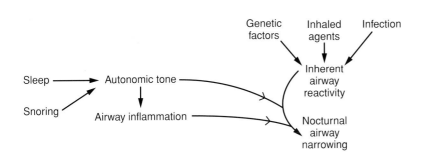

Figure 10.2
Diagram of the mechanisms of nocturnal asthma.

Clinical consequences

The main presentations are with cough, breathlessness, chest tightness or wheeze either disturbing sleep or causing problems first thing in the morning. These features can occur every day or, more usually, only when the patient's asthma is unstable. In some, the symptoms can be intractable but in most they are transient and respond to increased therapy. This symptom complex is usually accompanied by either a current or previous story of classical asthma during the daytime as well.

SLEEP

The major complaint of many patients with nocturnal asthma is about sleep disturbance and feeling sleepy by day. Sleep studies have confirmed sleep disruption with decreased sleep efficiency and increased intervening wakefulness and drowsiness.[48–50] This sleep disturbance probably causes the impaired cognitive performance found in patients with nocturnal asthma compared to age- and education-matched normal subjects.[50] Thus, the sleep problems could have a profound effect on the school and work performance of patients with nocturnal asthma.

During exacerbations of asthma, patients often have several consecutive nights when they get little sleep because of nocturnal symptoms. Even one night of sleep deprivation is enough to decrease ventilatory response by one-third,[51] and this reduction may be important, along with fatigue and continuing airway narrowing, in the development of hypoxaemia and hypercapnia in some patients with acute severe asthma.

HYPOXAEMIA

Patients with nocturnal asthma usually do not become severely hypoxaemic during sleep, but mild hypoxaemia is common.[48,49] Desaturation has been found to occur in some,[49,52] but not all[53] patients before they wake with wheeze. There have been no studies of oxygenation and sleep in patients with acute severe asthma.

NOCTURNAL ASTHMA ATTACKS

As a consequence of nocturnal airway narrowing, asthma attacks are more common at night than day, with increased presentations with attacks both to general practitioners and to emergency departments.[54] This timing is inconvenient to patients, their families and friends and to the medical staff whose assistance is required.

DEATHS

Although asthma deaths are uncommon, disproportionately more of these deaths occur by night than by day.[55] This excess nocturnal mortality is greater than occurs in the general population. These deaths could have many explanations, including the victim being unaware of the development of the attack because they were asleep and the inability of hypoxaemia, hypercapnia or increased airflow resistance to rapidly awaken them. Also, reluctance to seek help during the night could be a factor, although the fact that eight of 10 ventilatory arrests in asthmatics in hospital occurred at night suggests that delay in obtaining medical assistance is not the only factor.[56]

Diagnosis

A classical story in conjunction with evidence of asthma is usually sufficient. However, sometimes it is necessary to monitor peak expiratory flow rates for diagnosis as well as to guide therapy. Peak flow rates should be recorded a minimum of three times per day, on first waking, midday and at bedtime plus at any nocturnal wakings with symptoms. On each occasion, to increase accuracy, flow rates should be measured in triplicate and the highest reading taken. Overnight falls in peak flow rates of over 15 per cent in association with a suggestive history is diagnostic of nocturnal asthma.

Normally the diagnosis is clear but sometimes other causes of paroxysmal nocturnal dyspnoea will need to be excluded. These are:

- Pulmonary oedema – usually accompanied by history of heart disease, cardiomegaly and typical radiological features.
- Sleep apnoea/hypopnoea syndrome – brief episodes of choking, no wheeze.

Treatment

Symptomatic nocturnal airway narrowing is a sign of sub-optimal control of the patient's asthma. The new development of nocturnal symptoms in an asthma sufferer should always be regarded as a warning sign, which should trigger intensification of their therapy. It is important, however, to direct treatment at improvement of general asthma control and not merely to increase the use of bronchodilators which will act overnight. Thus the first line of therapy is to optimize use of prophylactic agents – usually inhaled steroids – and this is often sufficient.[57] Only when ideal control of both daytime symptoms and daytime peak flow rates is achieved should therapy be specifically targeted at the night-time.

Most patients with troublesome nocturnal asthma will treat themselves with an inhaled bronchodilator at bedtime. However, conventional inhaled beta$_2$-agonists only last about four hours, whereas nocturnal airway narrowing is mainly a problem late in the night. Inhaled atropine-like drugs tend to last for slightly longer and have the theoretical advantage of directly opposing the increase in parasympathetic tone which is a causative factor. Nevertheless, their role in the management of nocturnal asthma has proved relatively disappointing.

Newer, long-acting inhaled beta$_2$-agonists, such as salmeterol and formoterol, have actions lasting for at least 12 hours. Both have been shown to decrease symptoms and increase morning peak flow rates (Figure 10.3) in patients with nocturnal asthma.[58,59]

Salmeterol has also been found to improve sleep quality[58] by decreasing intervening wakefulness and drowsiness and increasing Stage 4 sleep. These agents represent a significant advance in the therapy of patients with troublesome nocturnal asthma.

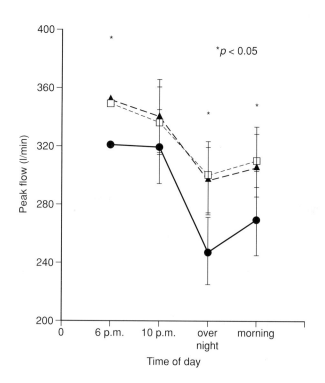

Figure 10.3
Effect of salmeterol 50 µgm bd (triangles) or 100 µgm bd (squares) in comparison to placebo MDI (circles) throughout the day in a randomized, double-blind trial in which each of 18 patients inhaled each agent twice daily for four weeks. (Data redrawn from Fitzpatrick (1990) Salmeterol in nocturnal asthma: a double blind, placebo controlled trial of a long acting inhaled beta$_2$ agonist. *BMJ*, 301, 1365–8, with permission from the BMJ Publishing Group.)

Oral sustained-release bronchodilators, such as theophyllines,[60] can also improve symptoms and morning peak flow rates. Once-daily dosage at bedtime is often sufficient[61] and minimizes daytime side-effects. Larger doses of theophylline can be given at night than during the day because absorption is slower.[62] It is unclear what effect theophylline therapy has on sleep quality. Earlier studies suggested sleep was impaired by theophyllines in asthmatics[60] but this has not been confirmed in normal subjects.[63]

There was no difference in sleep quality in asthmatics taking theophyllines in comparison to inhaled salmeterol.[64] This randomized study found no major differences between theophylline and salmeterol in the management of nocturnal asthma, with the minor benefits all favouring salmeterol including slightly fewer arousals from sleep, more nights without awakenings and better quality of life.[64] These differences were slight, so the major factors determining which agent to use should be patient preference and side-effects. Another randomized, controlled trial found that salmeterol was superior to oral sustained-release terbutaline in producing nights without wakening, higher morning peak flow rates and satisfaction with therapy.[65]

Physicians differ in their rank order of introducing high-dose inhaled steroids or long-acting bronchodilators. With recognition that long-term use of inhaled beta$_2$-agonist does not appear to carry hazard, these agents are increasingly being recommended before the dosage of inhaled steroids is increased.[66] Patients who do not respond to high-dose inhaled steroids plus bronchodilators may require treatment with oral steroids either for the short or long term.

In the small minority of patients who are known to be loud snorers, CPAP therapy should be tried if they do not readily respond to increased anti-asthma therapy[30] (Figure 10.4). It is also important to remember to check whether patients whose nocturnal asthma is proving difficult to control are loud snorers and have features of sleep apnoea.

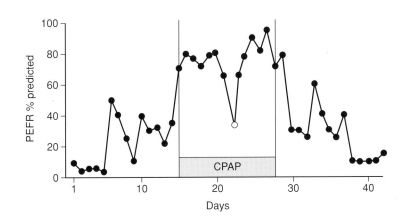

Figure 10.4
Peak expiratory flow rate (PEFR) at 0300 hours in an asthmatic subject with coincident OSAHS showing the marked improvement in peak flow with CPAP therapy (shaded area). The open symbol represents a night when CPAP was withdrawn. (Data redrawn from Chan.[30])

Conclusion

Nocturnal asthma causes significant inconvenience to large numbers of people. The development of inhaled long-acting bronchodilators has improved management.

References

1   Floyer J. (1698) *A Treatise on the Asthma.* London.
2   Turner-Warwick, M. (1984) Definition and recognition of nocturnal asthma, in P.J. Barnes, J. Levy (eds). *Nocturnal Asthma,* pp. 3–9. London: Royal Society of Medicine; International Congress and Symposium series. Number 73.
3   Turner-Warwick, M. (1989) Nocturnal asthma: a study in general practice. *J. R. Coll. Gen. Pract.,* **39**, 239–43.
4   Fitzpatrick, M.F., Martin, K., Fossey, E., Shapiro, C.M., Elton, R.A., Douglas, N.J. (1993) Snoring, asthma and sleep disturbance in Britain: a community-based survey. *Eur. Respir. J.,* **6**, 531–5.
5   Connolly, C.K. (1979) Diurnal rhythms in airway obstruction. *Br. J. Dis. Chest,* **73**, 357–66.
6   Kerr, H.D. (1973) Diurnal variation of respiratory function independent of air quality: experience with an environmentally controlled exposure chamber for human subjects. *Arch. Environ. Health,* **26**, 144–52.
7   Hetzel, M.R., Clark, T.J. (1980) Comparison of normal and asthmatic circadian rhythms in peak expiratory flow rate. *Thorax,* **35**, 732–8.
8   Hetzel, M.R., Clark, T.J. (1979) Does sleep cause nocturnal asthma? *Thorax,* **34**, 749–54.
9   Connolly, C.K. (1981) The effect of bronchodilators on diurnal rhythms in airway obstruction. *Br. J. Dis. Chest,* **75**, 197–203.
10 Catterall, J.R., Rhind, G.B., Stewart, I.C., Whyte, K.F., Shapiro, C.M., Douglas, N.J. (1986) Effect of sleep deprivation on overnight bronchoconstriction in nocturnal asthma. *Thorax,* **41**, 676–80.
11 Davies, R.J., Green, M., Schofield, N.M. (1976) Recurrent nocturnal asthma after exposure to grain dust. *Am. Rev. Respir. Dis.,* **114**, 1011–19.
12 Ryan, G., Latimer, K.M., Dolovich, J., Hargreave, F.E. (1982) Bronchial responsiveness to histamine: relationship to diurnal variation of peak flow rate, improvement after bronchodilator, and airway calibre. *Thorax,* **37**, 423–9.
13 Scherr, M.S., Peck, L.W. (1977) The effects of high efficiency air filtration system on nighttime asthma attacks. *W. V. Med. J.,* **73**, 144–8.

14   Platts-Mills, T.A., Mitchell, E.B. (1982) House dust mite avoidance. *Lancet*, **2**, 1334.

15   Platts-Mills, T.A., Vaughan, J.W., Carter, M.C., Woodfolk, J.A. (2000) The role of intervention in established allergy: Avoidance of indoor allergens in the treatment of chronic allergic disease. *J. Allergy Clin. Immunol.*, **106**, 787–804.

16   Chen, W.Y., Chai, H. (1982) Airway cooling and nocturnal asthma. *Chest*, **81**, 675–80.

17   Clark, T.J., Hetzel, M.R. (1977) Diurnal variation of asthma. *Br. J. Dis. Chest*, **71**, 87–92.

18   Whyte, K.F., Douglas, N.J. (1989) Posture and nocturnal asthma. *Thorax*, **44**, 579–81.

19   Cuttitta, G., Cibella, F., Visconti, A., Scichilone, N., Bellia, V., Bonsignore, G. (2000) Spontaneous gastroesophageal reflux and airway patency during the night in adult asthmatics. *Am. J. Respir. Crit. Care Med.*, **161**, 177–81.

20   Tan, W.C., Martin, R.J., Pandey, R., Ballard, R.D. (1990) Effects of spontaneous and simulated gastroesophageal reflux on sleeping asthmatics. *Am. Rev. Respir. Dis.*, **141**, 1394–9.

21   Hughes, D.M., Spier, S., Rivlin, J., Levison, H. (1983) Gastroesophageal reflux during sleep in asthmatic patients. *J. Pediatr.*, **102**, 666–72.

22   Martin, M.E., Grunstein, M.M., Larsen, G.L. (1982) The relationship of gastroesophageal reflux to nocturnal wheezing in children with asthma. *Ann. Allergy*, **49**, 318–22.

23   Ford, G.A., Oliver, P.S., Prior, J.S., Butland, R.J., Wilkinson, S.P. (1994) Omeprazole in the treatment of asthmatics with nocturnal symptoms and gastro-oesophageal reflux: a placebo-controlled crossover study. *Postgrad. Med. J.*, **70**, 350–4.

24   Kiljander, T.O., Salomaa, E.R., Hietanen, E.K., Terho, E.O. (1999) Gastroesophageal reflux in asthmatics: a double-blind, placebo-controlled crossover study with omeprazole. *Chest*, **116**, 1257–64.

25   Coughlan, J.L., Gibson, P.G., Henry, R.L. (2001) Medical treatment for reflux oesophagitis does not consistently improve asthma control: a systematic review. *Thorax*, **56**, 198–204.

26   De Vries, K., Goie, J., Booy-Nord, H., Orie, N.G.M. (1962) Changes during 24 hours in the lung function and histamine hyper-reactivity of the bronchial tree in asthmatic and bronchitic patients. *Int. Arch. Allergy*, **20**, 93–101.

27   Gervais, P., Reinberg, A., Gervais, C., Smolensky, M., DeFrance, O. (1977) Twenty-four-hour rhythm in the bronchial hyperreactivity to house dust in asthmatics. *J. Allergy Clin. Immunol.*, **59**, 207–13.

28   Heaton, R.W., Gillett, M.K., Snashall, P.D. (1988) Morning–evening

changes in airway responsiveness to methacholine in normal and asthmatic subjects: analysis using partial flow–volume curves. *Thorax*, **43**, 727–8.

29 Smolensky, M.H., Reinberg, A., Queng, J.T. (1981) The chronobiology and chronopharmacology of allergy. *Ann. Allergy*, 47, 234–52.

30 Chan, C.S., Woolcock, A.J., Sullivan, C.E. (1988) Nocturnal asthma: role of snoring and obstructive sleep apnea. *Am. Rev. Respir. Dis.*, **137**, 1502–4.

31 Baust, W., Bohnert, B. (1969) The regulation of heart rate during sleep. *Exp. Brain Res.*, 7, 169–80.

32 Morrison, J.F., Pearson, S.B., Dean, H.G. (1988) Parasympathetic nervous system in nocturnal asthma. *BMJ*, **296**, 1427–9.

33 Catterall, J.R., Rhind, G.B., Whyte, K.F., Shapiro, C.M., Douglas, N.J. (1988) Is nocturnal asthma caused by changes in airway cholinergic activity? *Thorax*, **43**, 720–4.

34 Hilton, M.F., Umali, M.U., Kres, S.B., Body, S., Czeisler, C.A., Wyatt, J.K. *et al.* (2000) Circadian variationof vagal and pulmonary function indices: a potential mechanism for nocturnal asthma. *Am. J. Resp. Crit. Care Med.*, **161**, A679.

35 Mackay, T.W., Fitzpatrick, M.F., Douglas, N.J. (1991) Non-adrenergic, non-cholinergic nervous system and overnight airway calibre in asthmatic and normal subjects. *Lancet*, **338**, 1289–92.

36 Mackay, T.W., Hulks, G., Douglas, N.J. (1998) Non-adrenergic, non-cholinergic function in the human airway. *Respir. Med.*, **92**, 461–6.

37 Corris, P.A., Dark, J.H. (1993) Aetiology of asthma: lessons from lung transplantation. *Lancet*, **341**, 1369–71.

38 Morrison, J.F., Teale, C., Pearson, S.B., Marshall, P., Dwyer, N.M., Jones, S. *et al.* (1990) Adrenaline and nocturnal asthma. *BMJ*, **301**, 473–6.

39 Jarjour, N.N., Busse, W.W., Calhoun, W.J. (1992) Enhanced production of oxygen radicals in nocturnal asthma. *Am. Rev. Respir. Dis.*, **146**, 905–11.

40 Kraft, M., Martin, R.J., Wilson, S., Djukanovic, R., Holgate, S.T. (1999) Lymphocyte and eosinophil influx into alveolar tissue in nocturnal asthma. *Am. J. Respir. Crit. Care Med.*, **159**, 228–34.

41 Mackay, T.W., Wallace, W.A., Howie, S.E., Brown, P.H., Greening, A.P., Church, M.K. *et al.* (1994) Role of inflammation in nocturnal asthma. *Thorax*, **49**, 257–62.

42 Martin, R.J., Cicutto, L.C., Smith, H.R., Ballard, R.D., Szefler, S.J. (1991) Airways inflammation in nocturnal asthma. *Am. Rev. Respir. Dis.*, **143**, 351–7.

43 ten Hacken, N.H., Postma, D.S., Bosma, F., Drok, G., Rutgers, B., Kraan, J. *et al.* (1993) Vascular adhesion molecules in nocturnal

asthma: a possible role for VCAM-1 in ongoing airway wall inflammation. *Clin. Exp. Allergy*, **28**, 1518–25.

44 Kraft, M., Striz, I., Georges, G., Umino, T., Takigawa, K., Rennard, S. *et al.* (1998) Expression of epithelial markers in nocturnal asthma. *J. Allergy Clin. Immunol.*, **102**, 376–81.

45 ten Hacken, N.H., Timens, W., Smith, M., Drok, G., Kraan, J., Postma, D.S. (1998) Increased peak expiratory flow variation in asthma: severe persistent increase but not nocturnal worsening of airway inflammation. *Eur. Respir. J.*, **12**, 546–50.

46 Jarjour, N.N., Busse, W.W. (1995) Cytokines in bronchoalveolar lavage fluid of patients with nocturnal asthma. *Am. J. Respir. Crit. Care Med.*, **152**, 1474–7.

47 Oosterhoff, Y., Kauffman, H.F., Rutgers, B., Zijlstra, F.J., Koeter, G.H., Postma, D.S. (1995) Inflammatory cell number and mediators in bronchoalveolar lavage fluid and peripheral blood in subjects with asthma with increased nocturnal airways narrowing. *J. Allergy Clin. Immunol.*, **96**, 219–29.

48 Catterall, J.R., Douglas, N.J., Calverley, P.M., Brash, H.M., Brezinova, V., Shapiro, C.M. *et al.* (1982) Irregular breathing and hypoxaemia during sleep in chronic stable asthma. *Lancet*, **1**, 301–4.

49 Montplaisir, J., Walsh, J., Malo, J.L. (1982) Nocturnal asthma: features of attacks, sleep and breathing patterns. *Am. Rev. Respir. Dis.*, **125**, 18–22.

50 Fitzpatrick, M.F., Engleman, H., Whyte, K.F., Deary, I.J., Shapiro, C.M., Douglas, N.J. (1991) Morbidity in nocturnal asthma: sleep quality and daytime cognitive performance. *Thorax*, **46**, 569–73.

51 White, D.P., Douglas, N.J., Pickett, C.K., Zwillich, C.W., Weil, J.V. (1983) Sleep deprivation and the control of ventilation. *Am. Rev. Respir. Dis.*, **128**, 984–6.

52 Deegan, P.C., McNicholas, W.T. (1994) Continuous non-invasive monitoring of evolving acute severe asthma during sleep. *Thorax*, **49**, 613–14.

53 Issa, F.G., Sullivan, C.E. (1985) Respiratory muscle activity and thoracoabdominal motion during acute episodes of asthma during sleep. *Am. Rev. Respir. Dis.*, **132**, 999–1004.

54 Horn, C.R., Clark, T.J., Cochrane, G.M. (1987) Is there a circadian variation in respiratory morbidity? *Br. J. Dis. Chest*, **81**, 248–51.

55 Douglas, N.J. (1985) Asthma at night. *Clin. Chest Med.*, **6**, 663–74.

56 Hetzel, M.R., Clark, T.J., Branthwaite, M.A. (1977) Asthma: analysis of sudden deaths and ventilatory arrests in hospital. *BMJ*, **1**, 808–11.

57 Horn, C.R., Clark, T.J., Cochrane, G.M. (1984) Inhaled therapy reduces morning dips in asthma. *Lancet*, **1**, 1143–5.

58 Fitzpatrick, M.F., Mackay, T., Driver, H., Douglas, N.J. (1990) Salmeterol in nocturnal asthma: a double blind, placebo controlled trial of a long acting inhaled beta$_2$ agonist. *BMJ*, **301**, 1365–8.

59 Maesen, F.P., Smeets, J.J., Gubbelmans, H.L., Zweers, P.G. (1990) Formoterol in the treatment of nocturnal asthma. *Chest*, **98**, 866–70.

60 Rhind, G.B., Connaughton, J.J., McFie, J., Douglas, N.J., Flenley, D.C. (1985) Sustained release choline theophyllinate in nocturnal asthma. *BMJ*, **291**, 1605–7.

61 Barnes, P.J., Greening, A.P., Neville, L., Timmers, J., Poole, G.W. (1982) Single-dose slow-release aminophylline at night prevents nocturnal asthma. *Lancet*, **1**, 299–301.

62 Scott, P.H., Tabachnik, E., MacLeod, S., Correia, J., Newth, C., Levison, H. (1981) Sustained-release theophylline for childhood asthma: evidence for circadian variation of theophylline pharmacokinetics. *J. Pediatr.*, **99**, 476–9.

63 Fitzpatrick, M.F., Engleman, H.M., Boellert, F., McHardy, R., Shapiro, C.M., Deary, I.J. *et al.* (1991) Effect of therapeutic theophylline levels on the sleep quality and daytime cognitive performance of normal subjects. *Am. Rev. Respir. Dis.*, **145**, 1355–8.

64 Selby, C., Engleman, H.M., Fitzpatrick, M.F., Sime, P.M., Mackay, T.W., Douglas, N.J. (1997) Inhaled salmeterol or oral theophylline in nocturnal asthma? *Am. J. Respir. Crit. Care Med.*, **155**, 104–8.

65 Brambilla, C., Chastang, C., Georges, D., Bertin, L. (1994) Salmeterol compared with slow-release terbutaline in nocturnal asthma. A multi-center, randomized, double-blind, double-dummy, sequential clinical trial. French Multicenter Study Group. *Allergy*, **49**, 421–6.

66 Greening, A.P., Ind, P.W., Northfield, M., Shaw, G. (1994) Added salmeterol versus higher-dose corticosteroid in asthma patients with symptoms on existing inhaled corticosteroid. *Lancet*, **344**, 219–24.

Sleep and medical conditions

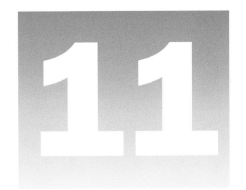

Many medical conditions are affected by sleep and, conversely, many may disturb sleep. The list is virtually endless as all conditions causing discomfort can impair sleep quality so this review is limited to a few. Those seeking further details are referred to major sleep textbooks such as Kryger, Roth and Dement.[1]

Cardiovascular disease

ANGINA

Sleep-related nocturnal angina was recorded in the eighteenth century and seems to occur mainly in REM sleep.[2,3] In patients with unstable angina about two-thirds of episodes happen between 10 pm and 8 am[4] (Figure 11.1). Patients with Prinzmetal's angina frequently experience symptoms during the night.

Figure 11.1
The circardian pattern of ischaemic activity, showing a significant night-time peak between 2200 and 0800 hours. (Data redrawn from Patel,[4] with permission.)
UA: unstable angina
Non Q: Non Q wave myocardial infarction

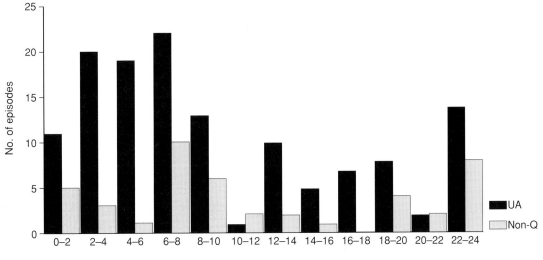

MYOCARDIAL INFARCTION

There is a peak in myocardial infarctions (MI) and sudden cardiac deaths between midnight and 0200 hours and a trough of MI frequency between 0300 and 0500 hours.[5] The late-night decrease may be related to decreased myocardial metabolic requirements during non-REM sleep.

CARDIAC ARRHYTHMIAS

Relative bradycardia is the norm during sleep as parasympathetic tone is increased.[6] In patients who have had myocardial infarctions there is evidence[7] of decreased dominance of the parasympathetic and increased sympathetic activity during sleep (Figure 11.2). This could predispose to increased risk of arrhythmias during sleep but it is contentious whether such an increased risk occurs.

Figure 11.2
Mean and SEM of the low-to high-frequency ratio (LF/HF) from spectral analysis of the RR interval during different sleep states in normal control subjects and patients post-myocardial infarction (post-MI). The ratios differ between patients and control subjects with higher LF/HF ratios during sleep in the patients, indicating increased sympathetic activity during sleep. (Data redrawn from Vanoli,[7] with permission.)

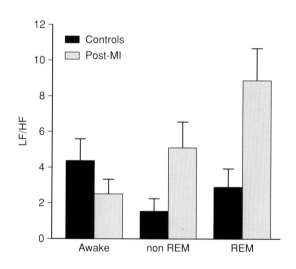

HYPERTENSION

Hypertensive subjects who do not show the normal fall of at least 10 per cent in blood pressure at night compared to the day are termed 'non-dippers'. Non-dippers are at increased risk of end organ damage, including left ventricular hypertrophy and cerebrovascular disease.[8] The reason for non-dipping presumably relates to disordered baroceptor function but this is not proven. Obstructive sleep apnoea/hypopnoea syndrome (OSAHS) is associated with marked surges in blood pressure with each arousal and so non-dipping is common in OSAHS, but this probably does not account for much of the non-dipping in the general hypertensive population. OSAHS is, however, a risk factor for hypertension, independent of obesity, gender, alcohol and other risk factors.[9,10]

CARDIAC FAILURE

Patients with severe left heart failure often have the cyclical breathing pattern of Cheyne–Stokes respiration, named after two Irish physicians who described it in 1818[11] and 1854,[12] respectively. This breathing pattern of cyclical hyperventilation followed by hypoventilation or apnoea does occur in wakefulness but is most prominent in stages 1 and 2 sleep,[13] and less so in slow wave or REM sleep. The recurrent arousals can contribute to the cyclical breathing pattern by repeatedly altering the ventilatory drive to breathing thus predisposing to a cyclical breathing pattern with a tendency to central apnoeas as the CO_2 levels fall below the apnoeic threshold. The presence of Cheyne–Stokes respiration is a strong independent predictor of mortality in patients with stable cardiac failure.[14] The cyclical breathing pattern is also associated with cyclical sleep disruption which may cause paroxysmal nocturnal dyspnoea, unrefreshing nocturnal sleep and daytime sleepiness.[15]

Treatment is by optimizing control of the cardiac failure with the addition of oxygen therapy.[16] If that does not suffice CPAP has been shown to be successful in some patients.[17] However, other centres have not been so successful[18] and there is no doubt that getting these patients to use CPAP is much more difficult than OSAHS patients. Newer therapies with intelligent ventilators designed to smooth out Cheyne–Stokes respiration remain to be adequately tested, although preliminary reports are encouraging.

> # Useful review
>
> - Naughton, M.T. (1998) Heart failure and central apnoea. *Sleep Medicine Reviews*, **2**, 105–16.

Cerebrovascular disease

Stroke occurs most commonly in the early morning after wakening, with a 49 per cent increase in stroke rate between 0600 and 1200 hours in a meta-analysis of 11,816 strokes[19] and a significantly lower frequency during the hours of sleep. However, there are several interactions between stroke and sleep.

Snoring is a risk factor for stroke[20] even when allowance is made for possible co-morbidities.[21] OSAHS is associated with hypertension[9,10] and thus it seems likely there is an independent causative association between OSAHS and stroke, although this has not been directly proved. Conversely, irregular breathing during sleep is very common after stroke with increased obstructive apnoeas and hypopnoeas in most patients,[22–25] especially in the first few weeks.[26] This may contribute to sleep disruption, daytime sleepiness and inattention which might impair recovery from stroke and even predispose to further stroke by increasing arterial blood pressure. This is an area of active study at present. Many patients may also have Cheyne–Stokes respiration after strokes with recurrent central apnoeas.

Sleepiness can occur after stroke or head injuries (*see* Chapter 4) and this can be independent of the occurrence of OSAHS. Somnolence can occur after unilateral or bilateral strokes affecting the para-median thalamus, mes-encephalon or rostral ascending reticular activating system among other areas.[27]

Insomnia is common after stroke and management is standard (*see* Chapter 6) with special attention being paid to trying to prevent sleep during the day, increasing exercise and ensuring exposure to daylight to entrain circadian rhythms of sleepiness. These are often difficult goals to achieve in practice, particularly in relatively immobile or institutionalized patients.

Stroke and cerebrovascular disease can also predispose to the development of REM sleep behavioural disorder (*see* Chapter 8). This is best treated with a benzodiazepine or REM sleep-suppressing antidepressant at bedtime (*see* Chapter 3).

Neuromuscular disease

Breathing problems during sleep are very common in patients with neuro-muscular problems. These may result either from inability to generate sufficient inspiratory pressure or failure to maintain upper airway patency during sleep.

Inspiratory pump failure during sleep results from the marked dependence on the diaphragm during REM sleep when intercostal activity is decreased due to the generalized hypotonia of postural muscles in REM sleep.[28,29] Thus, patients with bilateral diaphragmatic paralysis become severely hypoxaemic during REM sleep and patients with diaphragm weakness may become significantly more hypoxaemic than during wakefulness or non-REM sleep. This REM-related hypoventilation can contribute to the development of cardio-respiratory failure especially in those with co-existing lung disease. Such diaphragmatic weakness may be found in a wide range of neuromuscular diseases, including muscular dystrophies,[30,31] myotonic dystrophy, motor neurone disease,[32] myasthenia gravis, post-polio and Charcot–Marie–Tooth disease.[33] Patients with Duchenne muscular dystrophy often develop marked kyphoscoliosis which may result in inefficient diaphragmatic angle of action and consequences similar to diaphragm palsy.[34] Treatment of REM sleep-related hypoxaemia due to diaphragm malfunction is by nocturnal intermittent positive pressure ventilation (NIPPV) using a nasal or face mask. The usual indications for NIPPV are morning headache with documented associated carbon dioxide retention, ventilatory failure or marked daytime sleepiness. Patient compliance with this therapy is excellent.[35]

Upper airway dilating muscle failure can occur in myotonic dystrophy and in other neuromuscular conditions. These predispose to the development of OSAHS with all the classical symptoms (*see* Chapter 2). CPAP therapy can be useful.

Epilepsy

Sleep and epilepsy interact. In some epileptic patients seizures occur mainly or exclusively during sleep and in others awakening is associated with an increased likelihood of fits. Sleep-related epileptic activity is more common in non-REM sleep[36] and most common in slow wave sleep at least in temporal lobe epilepsy.[37] The increased frequency in non-REM sleep is believed to be a consequence of the neuronal synchronization in non-REM facilitating spread of epileptiform activity over the brain. This is compatible with the observation that temporal lobe epilepsy is more likely to become generalized during non-REM sleep.[38] In contrast, the desynchronized neuronal activity in REM sleep and wakefulness do not promote such progression.

Sleep deprivation promotes epileptic seizures. The diagnostic yield of routine EEGs can be significantly increased by overnight sleep deprivation.[39,40] Indeed, this technique has been recommended for patients in whom diagnostic difficulty is encountered.

Epilepsy may co-exist with sleep disorders. Some patients with both OSAHS and epilepsy gain significantly better control of their epilepsy once their OSAHS is treated.[41]

Obesity hypoventilation syndrome

Patients who are profoundly obese can have marked hypoventilation during sleep even in the absence of OSAHS. These patients may develop sustained daytime hypoxaemia and hypercapnia without having significant lung disease.

Very obese individuals have a restrictive pattern of lung function[42] with decreased compliance of the chest wall.[43] Lying down may further compromise respiration due to mass loading by abdominal contents both further decreasing lung volume and impairing diaphragm function. Sleep then worsens breathing more giving rise to recurrent desaturation and the 'obesity hypoventilation syndrome'. The diagnostic criteria are a BMI of more than 35 kg/m² with a raised arterial PCO_2 either during or immediately after sleep.[44]

All such patients should have detailed lung function tests to identify any lung disease and recording of their overnight breathing pattern to determine whether there is co-existing OSAHS. Sleep studies usually show hypoxaemia during sleep which is worst in REM sleep. If there is no OSAHS, treatment is by a combination of weight loss and nocturnal nasal IPPV.

Gastrointestinal disorders

Nocturnal gastrointestinal symptoms are common, although the relationships to sleep may be indirect.

GASTRO-OESOPHAGEAL REFLUX

Heartburn is common at night and is probably related to a combination of the horizontal position, slower oesophageal clearance of acid associated with decreased salivation – and thus decreased neutralization – and decreased swallows,[45] and slowed gastric emptying. Arousals from sleep promote oesophageal acid clearance and will thus decrease oesophagitis.

PEPTIC ULCER DISEASE

Basal gastric acid secretion is maximal around midnight,[46] although not directly related to sleep stage. Patients with duodenal ulcers have been shown to have impaired suppression of acid during the early hours of sleep.[47] This may explain why nocturnal dyspepsia is such a common feature of peptic ulcer disease.

Endocrine disorders

Many endocrine disorders are associated with OSAHS, although the reasons for the association vary.

ACROMEGALY

Around 60 per cent of people with acromegaly have sleep apnoea/hypopnoea[48] and sleepiness is a common feature of acromegaly. Although most have obstructive events, some studies have reported up to a third having mainly central apnoeas.

GROWTH HORMONE IN OSAHS

Patients with OSAHS have relatively low levels of growth hormone which presumably relates to the lack of REM sleep. Certainly, growth hormone levels return to normal with CPAP therapy[49] as sleep structure improves.

TESTOSTERONE TREATMENT

Hypogonadal males or normal women can develop OSAHS following treatment with testosterone. This only occurs in a minority of subjects but can be clinically important.[50] The mechanism may be increased tissue bulk in the neck, and perhaps increased muscle bulk may be an important factor.

PROGESTAGENS

Although the frequency of OSAHS in pre-menopausal women is relatively low, there is no good evidence that progestagens are protective and the difference may be age rather than hormonal.

HYPOTHYROIDISM

Several studies have found an increased frequency of OSAHS in patients with hypothyroidism[51,52] but the association has been challenged. The association is not strong enough to make screening for hypothyroidism cost-effective among all OSAHS patients[53,54] but thyroid function should be checked if there is any clinical suspicion of hypothyroidism.

DIABETES

The association between diabetes and OSAHS is largely, or perhaps entirely, due to associated obesity. Suggestions that diabetic autonomic neuropathy is associated with increased irregular breathing during sleep have been disputed.[55]

Renal disease

Patients with chronic renal failure receiving either haemo- or peritoneal dialysis have a high frequency of sleep complaints. Around 80 per cent report frequent nocturnal wakenings and 50 per cent daytime sleepiness. They have high frequencies of OSAHS[56,57] which will respond to CPAP. Central sleep apnoea can also occurs, but less often. Both the restless leg syndrome and periodic limb movement disorder (PLMD) are common[58] and can respond to L-dopa or other conventional therapies (*see* Chapter 8).

Pregnancy

Snoring is common during pregnancy affecting about 20 per cent,[59,60] but the mechanism is not clear. It may be due to upper airway narrowing resulting from the mass loading of the abdomen producing upper airway shortening and narrowing. There is some evidence that snoring and upper airway obstruction are more common in pre-eclampsia and that CPAP can contribute to a reduction in blood pressure.[61] The importance of these observations awaits clarification.

References

1 Kryger, Roth, Dement (2000) *Principles and Practice of Sleep Medicine.* Philadelphia: WB Saunders.
2 Nowlin, J.B., Troyer, W.G., Collins, W.S., Silverman, G., Nichols, C.R., McIntosh, H.D. *et al.* (1965) The association of nocturnal angina pectoris with dreaming. *Ann. Intern. Med.*, **63**, 1040–6.
3 Lichstein, E., Alosilla, C., Chadda, K.D., Gupta, P.K. (1977) Significance and treatment of nocturnal angina preceding myocardial infarction. *Am. Heart J.*, **93**, 723–6.
4 Patel, D.J., Knight, C.J., Holdright, D.R., Mulcahy, D., Clarke, D., Wright, C. *et al.* (1997) Pathophysiology of transient myocardial ischemia in acute coronary syndromes. Characterization by continuous ST-segment monitoring. *Circulation*, **95**, 1185–92.
5 Lavery, C.E., Mittleman, M.A., Cohen, M.C., Muller, J.E., Verrier, R.L. (1997) Nonuniform nighttime distribution of acute cardiac events: a possible effect of sleep states. *Circulation*, **96**, 3321–7.
6 Baust, W., Bohnert, B. (1969) The regulation of heart rate during sleep. *Exp. Brain Res.*, 7, 169–80.

7   Vanoli, E., Adamson, P.B., Ba, L., Pinna, G.D., Lazzara, R., Orr, W.C. (1995) Heart rate variability during specific sleep stages. A comparison of healthy subjects with patients after myocardial infarction. *Circulation*, **91**, 1918–22.

8   Parati, G., Pomidossi, G., Albini, F., Malaspina, D., Mancia, G. (1987) Relationship of 24-hour blood pressure mean and variability to severity of target-organ damage in hypertension. *J. Hypertens.*, **5**, 93–8.

9   Peppard, P.E., Young, T., Palta, M., Skatrud, J. (2000) Prospective study of the association between sleep-disordered breathing and hypertension. *N. Engl. J. Med.*, **342**, 1378–84.

10 Nieto, F.J., Young, T.B., Lind, B.K., Shahar, E., Samet, J.M., Redline, S. *et al.* (2000) Association of sleep-disordered breathing, sleep apnea, and hypertension in a large community-based study. Sleep Heart Health Study. *JAMA*, **283**, 1829–36.

11 Cheyne, J. (1818) A case of apoplexy in which the fleshy part of the heart was converted into fat. *Dublin Hosp. Rep.*, **2**, 216–23.

12 Stokes, W. (1854) *The Disease of the Heart and the Aorta*. Dublin: Hodges and Smith.

13 Hanly, P.J., Millar, T.W., Steljes, D.G., Baert, R., Frais, M.A., Kryger, M.H. (1989) Respiration and abnormal sleep in patients with congestive heart failure. *Chest*, **96**, 480–8.

14 Lanfranchi, P.A., Braghiroli, A., Bosimini, E., Mazzuero, G., Colombo, R., Donner, C.F. *et al.* (1999) Prognostic value of nocturnal Cheyne–Stokes respiration in chronic heart failure. *Circulation*, **99**, 1435–40.

15 Takasaki, Y., Orr, D., Popkin, J., Rutherford, R., Liu, P., Bradley, T.D. (1989) Effect of nasal continuous positive airway pressure on sleep apnea in congestive heart failure. *Am. Rev. Respir. Dis.*, **140**, 1578–84.

16 Hanly, P.J., Millar, T.W., Steljes, D.G., Baert, R., Frais, M.A., Kryger, M.H. (1989) The effect of oxygen on respiration and sleep in patients with congestive heart failure. *Ann. Intern. Med.*, **111**, 777–82.

17 Naughton, M.T., Liu, P.P., Bernard, D.C., Goldstein, R.S., Bradley, T.D. (1995) Treatment of congestive heart failure and Cheyne–Stokes respiration during sleep by continuous positive airway pressure. *Am. J. Respir. Crit. Care Med.*, **151**, 92–7.

18 Davies, R.J., Harrington, K.J., Ormerod, O.J., Stradling, J.R. (1993) Nasal continuous positive airway pressure in chronic heart failure with sleep-disordered breathing. *Am. Rev. Respir. Dis.*, **147**, 630–4.

19 Elliott, W.J. (1998) Circadian variation in the timing of stroke onset: a meta-analysis. *Stroke*, **29**, 992–6.

20 Spriggs, D.A., French, J.M., Murdy, J.M., Curless, R.H., Bates, D., James, O.F. (1992) Snoring increases the risk of stroke and adversely affects prognosis. *Q. J. Med.*, **83**, 555–62.

21 Waller, P.C., Bhopal, R.S. (1989) Is snoring a cause of vascular disease? An epidemiological review. *Lancet*, **1**, 143–6.

22 Good, D.C., Henkle, J.Q., Gelber, D., Welsh, J., Verhulst, S. (1996) Sleep-disordered breathing and poor functional outcome after stroke. *Stroke*, **27**, 252–9.

23 Bassetti, C., Aldrich, M.S., Chervin, R.D., Quint, D. (1996) Sleep apnea in patients with transient ischemic attack and stroke: a prospective study of 59 patients. *Neurology*, **47**, 1167–73.

24 Bassetti, C., Aldrich, M.S. (1999) Sleep apnea in acute cerebrovascular diseases: final report on 128 patients. *Sleep*, **22**, 217–23.

25 Dyken, M.E., Somers, V.K., Yamada, T., Ren, Z.Y., Zimmerman, M.B. (1996) Investigating the relationship between stroke and obstructive sleep apnea. *Stroke*, **27**, 401–7.

26 Parra, O., Arboix, A., Bechich, S., Garcia-Eroles, L., Montserrat, J.M., Lopez, J.A. *et al.* (2000) Time course of sleep-related breathing disorders in first-ever stroke or transient ischemic attack. *Am. J. Respir. Crit. Care Med.*, **161**, 375–80.

27 Bassetti, C., Mathis, J., Gugger, M., Lovblad, K.O., Hess, C.W. (1996) Hypersomnia following paramedian thalamic stroke: a report of 12 patients. *Ann. Neurol.*, **39**, 471–80.

28 Jouvet, M., Michel, F. (1959) Correlations electromyographiques du sommeil chez le chat decortique et mesencephalique chronique. *C. R. Soc. Biol.*, **153**, 422.

29 Morales, F.R., Chase, M.H. (1978) Intracellular recording of lumbar motoneuron membrane potential during sleep and wakefulness. *Exp. Neurol.*, **62**, 821–7.

30 Phillips, M.F., Smith, P.E., Carroll, N., Edwards, R.H., Calverley, P.M. (1999) Nocturnal oxygenation and prognosis in Duchenne muscular dystrophy. *Am. J. Respir. Crit. Care Med.*, **160**, 198–202.

31 Skatrud, J., Iber, C., McHugh, W., Rasmussen, H., Nichols, D. (1980) Determinants of hypoventilation during wakefulness and sleep in diaphragmatic paralysis. *Am. Rev. Respir. Dis.*, **121**, 587–93.

32 Arnulf, I., Similowski, T., Salachas, F., Garma, L., Mehiri, S., Attali, V. *et al.* (2000) Sleep disorders and diaphragmatic function in patients with amyotrophic lateral sclerosis. *Am. J. Respir. Crit. Care Med.*, **161**, 849–56.

33 Chan, C.K., Mohsenin, V., Loke, J., Virgulto, J., Sipski, M.L., Ferranti, R. (1987) Diaphragmatic dysfunction in siblings with hereditary motor and sensory neuropathy (Charcot–Marie–Tooth disease). *Chest*, **91**, 567–70.

34 Smith, P.E., Calverley, P.M., Edwards, R.H., Evans, G.A., Campbell, E.J. (1987) Practical problems in the respiratory care of patients with muscular dystrophy. *N. Engl. J. Med.*, **316**, 1197–205.

35   Simonds, A.K., Elliott, M.W. (1995) Outcome of domiciliary nasal intermittent positive pressure ventilation in restrictive and obstructive disorders. *Thorax*, **50**, 604–9.

36   Malow, B.A., Kushwaha, R., Lin, X., Morton, K.J., Aldrich, M.S. (1997) Relationship of interictal epileptiform discharges to sleep depth in partial epilepsy. *Electroencephalogr. Clin. Neurophysiol.*, **102**, 20–6.

37   Malow, B.A., Lin, X., Kushwaha, R., Aldrich, M.S. (1998) Interictal spiking increases with sleep depth in temporal lobe epilepsy. *Epilepsia*, **39**, 1309–16.

38   Bazil, C.W., Walczak, T.S. (1997) Effects of sleep and sleep stage on epileptic and nonepileptic seizures. *Epilepsia*, **38**, 56–62.

39   Pratt, K.L., Mattson, R.H., Weikers, N.J., Williams, R. (1968) EEG activation of epileptics following sleep deprivation: a prospective study of 114 cases. *Electroencephalogr. Clin. Neurophysiol.*, **24**, 11–15.

40   Molaie, M., Cruz, A. (1988) The effect of sleep deprivation on the rate of focal interictal epileptiform discharges. *Electroencephalogr. Clin. Neurophysiol.*, **70**, 288–92.

41   Vaughn, B.V., D'Cruz, O.F., Beach, R., Messenheimer, J.A. (1996) Improvement of epileptic seizure control with treatment of obstructive sleep apnoea. *Seizure*, **5**, 73–8.

42   Thomas, P.S., Cowen, E.R., Hulands, G., Milledge, J.S. (1989) Respiratory function in the morbidly obese before and after weight loss. *Thorax*, **44**, 382–6.

43   Naimark, A., Cherniack, R.M. (1960) Compliance of the respiratory system in health and obesity. *J. Appl. Physiol.*, **15**, 377–82.

44   American Sleep Disorders Association. (1999) Sleep-related breathing disorders in adults: recommendations for syndrome definition and measurement techniques in clinical research. The Report of an American Academy of Sleep Medicine Task Force. *Sleep*, **22**, 667–89.

45   Orr, W.C., Johnson, L.F., Robinson, M.G. (1984) Effect of sleep on swallowing, esophageal peristalsis, and acid clearance. *Gastroenterology*, **86**, 814–19.

46   Feldman, M., Richardson, C.T. (1986) Total 24-hour gastric acid secretion in patients with duodenal ulcer. Comparison with normal subjects and effects of cimetidine and parietal cell vagotomy. *Gastroenterology*, **90**, 540–4.

47   Orr, W.C., Hall, W.H., Stahl, M.L., Durkin, M.G., Whitsett, T.L. (1976) Sleep patterns and gastric acid secretion in duodenal ucler disease. *Arch. Intern. Med.*, **136**, 655–60.

48   Grunstein, R.R., Ho, K.Y., Sullivan, C.E. (1991) Sleep apnea in acromegaly. *Ann. Intern. Med.*, **115**, 527–32.

49   Grunstein, R.R. (1996) Metabolic aspects of sleep apnea. *Sleep*, **19**, S218–S220.

50 Schneider, B.K., Pickett, C.K., Zwillich, C.W., Weil, J.V., McDermott, M.T., Santen, R.J. *et al.* (1986) Influence of testosterone on breathing during sleep. *J. Appl. Physiol.*, **61**, 618–23.

51 Grunstein, R.R., Sullivan, C.E. (1988) Sleep apnea and hypothyroidism: mechanisms and management. *Am. J. Med.*, **85**, 775–9.

52 Rajagopal, K.R., Abbrecht, P.H., Derderian, S.S., Pickett, C., Hofeldt, F., Tellis, C.J. *et al.* (1984) Obstructive sleep apnea in hypothyroidism. *Ann. Intern. Med.*, **101**, 491–4.

53 Skjodt, N.M., Atkar, R., Easton, P.A. (1999) Screening for hypothyroidism in sleep apnea. *Am. J. Respir. Crit. Care Med.*, **160**, 732–5.

54 Lin, C.C., Tsan, K.W., Chen, P.J. (1992) The relationship between sleep apnea syndrome and hypothyroidism. *Chest*, **102**, 1663–7.

55 Catterall, J.R., Calverley, P.M., Ewing, D.J., Shapiro, C.M., Clarke, B.F., Douglas, N.J. (1984) Breathing, sleep, and diabetic autonomic neuropathy. *Diabetes*, **33**, 1025–7.

56 Hallett, M., Burden, S., Stewart, D., Mahony, J., Farrell, P. (1995) Sleep apnea in end-stage renal disease patients on hemodialysis and continuous ambulatory peritoneal dialysis. *ASAIO J.*, **41**, M435–M441.

57 Stepanski, E., Faber, M., Zorick, F., Basner, R., Roth, T. (1995) Sleep disorders in patients on continuous ambulatory peritoneal dialysis. *J. Am. Soc. Nephrol.*, **6**, 192–7.

58 Winkelman, J.W., Chertow, G.M., Lazarus, J.M. (1996) Restless legs syndrome in end-stage renal disease. *Am. J. Kidney Dis.*, **28**, 372–8.

59 Loube, D.I., Poceta, J.S., Morales, M.C., Peacock, M.D., Mitler, M.M. (1996) Self-reported snoring in pregnancy. Association with fetal outcome. *Chest*, **109**, 885–9.

60 Franklin, K.A., Holmgren, P.A., Jonsson, F., Poromaa, N., Stenlund, H., Svanborg, E. (2000) Snoring, pregnancy-induced hypertension, and growth retardation of the fetus. *Chest*, **117**, 137–41.

61 Edwards, N., Blyton, D.M., Kirjavainen, T., Kesby, G.J., Sullivan, C.E. (2000) Nasal continuous positive airway pressure reduces sleep-induced blood pressure increments in preeclampsia. *Am. J. Respir. Crit. Care Med.*, **162**, 252–7.

Index